GETTING PREGNANT *Naturally*

GETTING PREGNANT *Naturally*

Healthy Choices to Boost Your Chances of Conceiving without Fertility Drugs

WINIFRED CONKLING

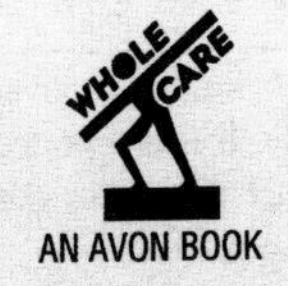

AN AVON BOOK

AVON BOOKS, INC.
1350 Avenue of the Americas
New York, New York 10019

Interior design by Rhea Braunstein
Published by arrangement with the author
ISBN: 0-380-79633-3
www.avonbooks.com/wholecare

Library of Congress Cataloging in Publication Data:

Conkling, Winifred.
Getting pregnant naturally : healthy choices to boost your chances of conceiving without fertility drugs / Winifred Conkling.
p. cm.
Includes bibliographical references.
1. Conception. 2. Fertility, Human.
3. Infertility—Alternative treatment. I. Title.
RG133.C64 1999 98-45199
618.2—dc21 CIP

First WholeCare Printing: June 1999
First Avon Books Trade Paperback Printing: February 1999

Printed in the U.S.A.

OPM 10 9 8 7 6 5 4

For Hannah and Ella

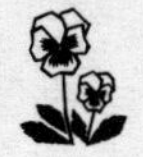

Note to the Reader

This book is not intended to take the place of advice from a trained medical professional. It was written to provide alternative methods for increasing fertility before turning to fertility drugs. Neither the publisher nor the author take any responsibility for the consequences of any treatment or actions mentioned in this book; they cannot guarantee that the methods described in these pages will result in pregnancy achievement for every couple. While every effort has been made to provide the most accurate and updated information, the publisher and author cannot be responsible for any errors, omissions, or dated material.

Contents

Introduction

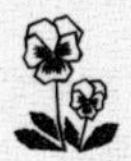

I don't like the word "infertility"; it leaves no room for hope, even though many couples who have trouble conceiving go on to have children. I have known women with ovulation disorders and damaged tubes who became pregnant; I have known men with one-sided varicoceles and low sperm counts who have impregnated their wives. Instead of using the word "infertile," I prefer to use the term "impaired fertility." I have worked with hundreds of couples with impaired fertility, and I know that there are many things couples can do to enhance their chances of conceiving a child.

Human reproduction is an inexact science; most people shift back and forth between periods of fertility and infertility as their bodies pass through various hormonal stages and respond to physical and emotional stresses.

Our hormones—and our fertility—change in response to age, diet, and nutrition, and exercise and lifestyle, among other factors. Some of these factors we can control, others we cannot.

When it comes to getting pregnant, it's up to you to make the most of each month. It's up to you to eat right, to rest, and to make healthy choices in your life. It's up to you to listen to your body; nobody knows your body better than you do. You must learn to recognize when something feels "off" so that you can follow up with a doctor.

If you are a man, it's up to you to protect your sperm. Most men don't realize that it takes almost three months to produce sperm, so that what you do today will affect your sperm months later. If you are a woman, it's up to you to learn how to chart your fertility so that you can better time intercourse to coincide with ovulation. A simple temperature chart can also help you detect common fertility problems, such as a luteal phase defect. In many cases, no single thing you do or don't do determines your fertility. It is the cumulative effect of a number of little things that can either enhance or impair your fertility. This is why you should do what you can to get pregnant naturally before you rush off to consult a reproductive endocrinologist.

The advice offered in this book can help you increase

your chances of conceiving a child. If you remain childless after a year, you may need to work with a fertility specialist. Of course, you may do everything right and still end up without a biological child.

I spent nine years trying to get pregnant, and I tried everything you can imagine. That's why I never ask anyone I meet, "How many children do you have?" I remember what a difficult question that was to answer when my husband and I were trying desperately to conceive.

I am now the mother of two adopted children. Once I accepted that my body was not going to reproduce and that my husband and I were not going to build a family the way that we had hoped, dreamed, and planned, I realized that adoption offered another option. While adoption was my second choice, it was *not* second-best. I have been blessed with two wonderful children. I am a mother. My husband and I have built our family. I have everything but a pregnancy story. Best of luck to those of you entering this journey.

ILENE STARGOT
Founder and Executive Director
National Infertility Network Exchange (NINE)

1

Infertile or Subfertile? An Overview

It's ironic: When couples don't want to have a baby, they assume that they are fertile and put a lot of energy into preventing pregnancy. Then, when they decide it's time to start a family, they suddenly appreciate how difficult it actually is to conceive a child.

Getting pregnant requires exquisite timing, a balanced hormonal system, good general health—and a measure of good fortune. A woman's endocrine system must release precise levels of hormones at specific times during her menstrual cycle. Her ovaries must produce and release at least one mature and healthy egg follicle, and that egg must be able to make its way through the Fallopian tubes toward a welcoming uterus. A man's reproductive system must produce semen containing an abundant supply of healthy sperm ready to swim eagerly toward the intended target. The woman's cervix must produce enough mucus to protect the sperm and hurry them into the uterus and Fallopian tubes. Once the egg and sperm have been united, the thickened uterine lining must be responsive and ready to nourish the fertilized egg after it has implanted.

A single missed cue or minor glitch, and the system doesn't work. Considering the complexities, it's no wonder that a healthy and fertile couple stands only a 20 percent chance of conceiving a child in any given month. It also explains why more than 5 million Americans of childbearing age are considered technically infertile, meaning they have tried to conceive a child for one year or more without success.

But there is hope. As many as half of all infertile couples do go on to get pregnant and have healthy babies. These couples could more accurately be defined as *subfertile*. They may not suffer from a physical problem that prevents conception, but it may take them longer than one year to become pregnant. For these couples, the stork may arrive sooner if Mother Nature is offered a little extra help.

UNDERSTANDING INFERTILITY

Most couples who want to have children are successful—some sooner, some later. Typically, half of the couples who decide to stop using contraception will conceive within three to five months, and about 85 percent of the couples will conceive within a year. However, that leaves 15 percent—or roughly one out of every six couples—who will experience fertility problems.

Impaired fertility has many causes. For about 35 to 40 percent of couples, the problem lies within the woman; for another 35 to 40 percent, the problem lies within the man; and in the rest, both partners have a problem or the cause is unknown.

Among women, hormonal imbalance is the most common cause of infertility. Other possible causes include scarring or obstruction of the Fallopian tubes, an allergic reaction to sperm, endometriosis, hostile cervical mucus, chromosomal abnormalities, a prolapsed uterus, fibroids, or physical injury to reproductive organs, among other causes. And, of course, age plays a significant role: A woman's fertility peaks in her mid-twenties; her fertility declines gradually until age thirty, and then begins to fall off more rapidly. Many women remain fertile into their forties, but conception becomes more difficult with each passing year.

Among men, abnormal sperm—either low sperm count or inferior sperm quality—is to blame for most fertility problems. It may take only one sperm to fertilize an egg, but the average ejaculation contains between 40 million and 150 million sperm. Most of these sperm don't stand a fighting chance of getting within striking distance of the awaiting egg; some 80 to 90 percent of them are killed off by vaginal fluids. Due to this intense screening process, men who ejaculate fewer than 60 million sperm may have difficulty impregnating their partners. In medical terminology, oligospermia means low sperm count and azoospermia means the absence of living sperm in the semen.

Not surprisingly, the number of sperm in an ejaculate and the degree of fertility are strongly correlated. But even men with low sperm counts can impregnate their partners. In fact, studies at fertility clinics have found that 52 percent of men whose sperm counts were below 10 million per milliliter of ejaculate achieved pregnancy, as did 40 percent of those with sperm counts as low as 5 million per milliliter of ejaculate.

Numbers count, but when it comes to fertility, sperm quality is even more important than quantity. A man can have a high number of sperm, but if a majority of them are abnormally shaped or poor swimmers, he can have a harder time becoming a father than a man with fewer sperm of a higher quality. Sperm quality is based on several factors, including motility (how fast and straight the sperm swims) and morphology (sperm size and shape). At least 60 percent of the sperm should be normal in appearance and motility. The quality of the seminal fluid—its volume and viscosity or stickiness—also plays an important role. Problems with sperm can stem from a number of causes, including a varicocele (a varicose vein in the scrotum), prostate infections, ductal obstructions, ejaculatory dysfunction, mumps, alcohol use, nicotine, illness, or excessive fatigue.

Many couples experience periods of infertility that come and go for no apparent reason. Approximately 25 percent of women have reported episodes of infertility at some point during their reproductive lives. In many cases, a couple may not know they are experiencing impaired fertility because they are not trying to get pregnant at that time. This ongoing fluctuation between periods of fertility and infertility may help to explain why each month approximately 3 percent of couples with unexplained infertility suddenly conceive on their own.

Subfertile couples may benefit from experimenting with the fertility-enhancing natural remedies and practices suggested in this book. Of course, fertility drugs

When to Get Help

If you and your partner have had intercourse without using contraception twice a week for a year without becoming pregnant, it's time to consider consulting a reproductive endocrinologist for counseling, as well as a urologist specializing in male-factor infertility. In addition, you should see a physician before the one-year mark if one of the following circumstances exist:

* If a woman is over age forty.
* If a woman is over age thirty-five and has not conceived after six months of regular unprotected intercourse.
* If either partner may have scarring or damage to reproductive organs because of infections or sexually transmitted diseases.
* If a woman has irregular periods or no periods at all.
* If a woman has used or is using an intrauterine device (IUD).
* If a woman has a history of endometriosis, pelvic infections, abdominal or urinary tract surgery, polycystic ovarian syndrome, or exposure to toxic chemicals or radiation.

- If a man has a history of mumps, measles, very high fevers, or exposure to toxic chemicals or radiation.
- If either partner is the child of a mother who took the synthetic estrogen diethylstilbestrol (DES) during pregnancy to prevent miscarriage. DES daughters often suffer from a range of reproductive problems; DES sons may have low sperm counts and other sperm anomalies.

and assisted reproductive technologies can offer hope to couples with serious reproductive problems, but most subfertile couples would do well to begin with simple, natural methods of enhancing their fertility. In many cases, these low-tech treatments will work and a couple can avoid turning to expensive, invasive, and stressful high-tech fertility treatments.

MILESTONES TO REMEMBER

- 1978: The world's first "test-tube baby," Louise Brown of Great Britain, was born.
- 1981: The first American test-tube baby, Elizabeth Jordan Carr, was born in Norfolk, Virginia.
- Mid-1980s: Surrogate mother Mary Beth Whitehead fought to maintain custody of the infant "Baby M," to whom she gave birth under contract with another couple.
- 1992: A sixty-two-year-old Sicilian widow became pregnant through artificial insemination with sperm that had been collected from her husband and frozen before he died.
- 1992: A fifty-three-year-old California grandmother gave birth to twin girls for her daughter. The babies were conceived in a petri dish using sperm from her son-in-law and eggs donated by a twenty-year-old woman.
- 1993: Several grandmothers gave birth to their own grandchildren, using eggs provided by their daughters and sperm from their sons-in-law.

2

Sex and Sexuality: The Birds and the Bees for Grown-ups

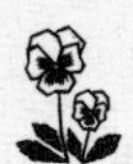

Timing is everything—at least when it comes to getting pregnant. To conceive a child, you and your partner must have intercourse within a very narrow window of time. An egg is fertile for only six to twenty-four hours after ovulation; after that time it begins to disintegrate. Understanding your reproductive system and how it works can help you time intercourse to maximize your chances of conceiving each month.

While the mechanics of intercourse may seem self-evident, certain practical issues can affect your fertility. Your creativity in the bedroom (or wherever) can increase—or decrease—your odds of conception. In other words, it's not just what you do, but how you do it. The following tips can help you get the timing down to a science—and help with some of the practical issues, too.

HERS

Get to Know Your Menstrual Cycle

As you know, to become pregnant you must have intercourse near the time of ovulation. The tough part, of course, is determining exactly when you ovulate. If you have been blessed with a consistent, predictable menstrual cycle, you can use the "calendar method." This method involves keeping track of the length of your menstrual cycle, then calculating when you are most likely to release an egg. If all your hormones are in balance, you probably ovulate approximately fourteen days before the first day of your next menstrual period. That makes it relatively easy to make an educated guess of the approximate date of ovulation.

To estimate your date of ovulation, take the length of your cycle and subtract fourteen days. For example, if you have a twenty-eight-day cycle, you ovulate on day fourteen (twenty-eight minus fourteen). If you have a thirty-five-day cycle, you ovulate on day twenty-one (thirty-five minus fourteen), and if you have a twenty-one-day cycle, you ovulate on day seven (twenty-one minus fourteen).

Chart your menstrual cycle for three months to form a baseline or average length of your cycle. The typical cycle ranges from twenty-four to thirty-six days, so don't get hung up on the "average" twenty-eight-day cycle.

Once you determine your approximate ovulation date, have intercourse every other day for five days before the target date and three days after. If you have intercourse every other day during this time, you will probably include your fertile time.

Monitor Your Cervical Mucus

Your cervical mucus doesn't lie: Once you become acquainted with its changes in texture and volume throughout your menstrual cycle, you may become adept at reading this crucial fertility marker.

Your cervical mucus changes in response to fluctuations in the level of estrogen in your body. During the first half of your cycle, the egg matures within the ovarian follicle and the body releases increasing amounts of estrogen. This estrogen helps thicken the lining of the uterus, preparing it for implantation of the fertilized egg. The hormonal changes also create the fertile cervical mucus, which helps the sperm reach the uterus and Fallopian tubes. The fertile mucus provides a protective alkaline medium for the sperm to travel through the vagina. You want to have intercourse during the time the fertile mucus is present.

After the estrogen has peaked (at ovulation), the progesterone levels surge, prompting a change in the cervical mucus, often in as little as a couple of hours. At this point, your chances of conception have passed.

Fertile mucus is noticeably different from mucus at other phases of your menstrual cycle: It is slick, transparent, gelatinous, and stringy. It is stretchy; in fact, you can rub it between two fingers and stretch it for an inch or more (nonfertile mucus does not stretch). When fertile mucus dries in the crotch of your panties, it may feel stiff and appear white or yellowish. (Some women mistakenly believe that they have a vaginal yeast infection or they have been remiss in their personal hygiene during this phase of their cycle, but this discharge is perfectly normal.)

Please note that you may not be able to use the cervical mucus test if you are taking birth control pills (or for at least two months after you stop taking them). Also be aware that bathing, showering, swimming, and unprotected intercourse can temporarily alter your mucus, so check your mucus before these activities or several hours after you're finished.

As a woman ages, she produces less fertile mucus. Twenty-something women often have two to four days of fertile mucus, while thirty-something women may have one day or less. The older you get, the more important it is for you to learn to recognize your fertile days so that you can take maximum advantage of them.

MEET YOUR MUCUS

- *Early in your cycle*: Your vagina will be dry with little or no cervical mucus.
- *As ovulation approaches*: A few days before ovulation your mucus flow will increase and become creamy, white, and wet. Begin having intercourse every forty-eight hours during this phase.
- *Fertile mucus at ovulation*: Your mucus will become thin, slippery, stretchy, and clear; it will resemble the appearance and consistency of egg white. You want to strive to have intercourse during the time you have fertile mucus.
- *After ovulation*: Immediately following ovulation your mucus will turn sticky, much like the consistency of rubber cement. After two or three days, it will become dry, until the cycle starts again.

Take Your Temperature

You can learn a lot about your body by using a thermometer. By keeping track of your basal body temperature—your temperature in the morning before you get out of bed—you can learn to approximate the time of ovulation and when in your cycle you will be most fertile. (Unfortunately, when monitoring the ever-changing cycle of fertility, we deal with approximations, not predictions.)

First, get a thermometer, a piece of paper, and a pen or pencil to record your temperature; keep these items by the side of the bed. To get an accurate reading, you're going to need to take your temperature *first* thing in the morning—meaning before you sit up in bed, before you go to the bathroom, before you say good morning to your spouse, before you talk to anyone on the phone.

Some women take their temperature rectally for a more accurate reading, but an oral thermometer should be sufficient in most cases. You may want to buy a basal body temperature thermometer, designed to make it easier to read the temperature to the tenth of a degree. These thermometers usually come with a preprinted chart and directions for monitoring your temperature. They are available in most drugstores and usually cost less than $10.

Try to take your temperature after at least three hours of consecutive sleep and at the same time each day, plus or minus an hour or so. Keep in mind that every extra half-hour you snooze your body temperature will rise by about one-tenth of a degree.

Most women report a slight drop in their temperature just before ovulation (when the levels of estrogen increase to release the egg during the next few days). A day or two later, they note a sharp rise of 0.5 to 1 point when the egg is released (when the levels of heat-producing progesterone increase). By the time the temperature spikes—usually to over 98 degrees, though it may go to 99 degrees or higher in some women—ovulation has already occurred.

This temperature shift—and ovulation—usually occur at fourteen days into your menstrual cycle, or about day fourteen of a twenty-eight-day cycle. The morning temperature then should remain elevated for the second half of the menstrual cycle (the luteal phase), dropping slightly just before menstruation when the cycle starts over again.

To maximize your chances of conception, have intercourse every other day for two to four days before you anticipate the shift in temperature (and ovulation), as well as two to four days after your temperature rises. (If you chart your temperature for several months, you will recognize your personal ovulation pattern and become more adept at detecting when ovulation should occur.)

Normal body temperatures vary from person to person, but it is the change in temperature, not the temperature itself, that is important in measuring fertility. You may have a hormonal imbalance and should consult a doctor if your temperature remains the same throughout your cycle (you may not be releasing an egg) or if your temperature tapers off during the second half of your cycle (you may not have sufficient hormonal support to produce a mature egg). If your temperature remains elevated for more than two weeks after ovulation, you may be pregnant!

Note Changes in Your Cervix

You can learn to recognize the approach of ovulation by learning to recognize the changes in your cervix as ovulation approaches. If you want additional information on how to detect ovulation, take time to feel your cervix throughout the month so that you can learn to appreciate the subtle but important changes that occur during your menstrual cycle:

- During your menstrual period, your cervix should be easy to touch with the tip of a finger inserted into the vagina. The area at the opening of the cervix should feel soft and opened wide to allow the uterine lining to escape.
- After the bleeding stops, your cervix should feel firm and tightly closed; some say it feels like the tip of a nose. If you have not delivered a child vaginally, the opening of the cervix may feel like a dimple or pointed impression. If you have had a child vaginally, the opening may feel wider.
- As the body prepares for ovulation, the cervix will

rise or move away from the vaginal opening. (You will have to insert your finger deeper into your vagina to feel it.) The cervical opening should feel softer and wider, to allow the sperm to enter the uterus and fertilize the ripened egg.

- After ovulation, the cervix lowers and grows firmer, and the opening closes tightly to prevent sperm from entering the uterus since conception can no longer occur.

Try an Ovulation Predictor Test

If you don't trust yourself to read your body's ovulation warning signs, you can pick up an ovulation predictor test kit at almost any pharmacy or grocery store for about $20. This test looks for the surge in luteinizing hormone (LH) that occurs just before ovulation. (The rise in LH actually triggers the release of the egg from the ovary.) Ovulation should take place twelve to thirty-six hours after the test is positive.

The kits are relatively easy to use and tend to be quite accurate—as long as you follow the directions. However, keep in mind that the test does not guarantee that ovulation has taken place. Some women, especially those with premature ovarian failure or those over age forty or approaching menopause, sometimes have LH surges that are not followed by the release of an egg. If you want some assurance that you are identifying your time of ovulation accurately, give an ovulation predictor kit a try for a month or two, but don't rely on this test if your infertility continues for several months longer.

Stay on Your Back for Twenty to Thirty Minutes After Intercourse

It takes about twenty minutes or so for the sperm to work their way through the cervical mucus and up to the Fallopian tubes in search of the prized egg. Staying horizontal won't guarantee success, but it can help minimize the risk of sperm leakage from the vagina—and it certainly can't hurt. Plan ahead and have a book, music, or the television remote nearby to help pass the time, or close your eyes and take a nap.

Don't Douche

Your vagina can keep itself clean, so there is no medical or hygienic reason to douche. Douching with commercial products can disrupt the natural pH of the vagina, possibly damaging or destroying sperm.

Even douching with plain water isn't good for you: It has been linked to an increased incidence of ectopic pregnancy and pelvic inflammatory disease. A recent study conducted by researchers from Emory University in Atlanta and the Federal Centers for Disease Control and Prevention found that women who douched were almost four times as likely as those who had not to develop an ectopic pregnancy. The longer a woman douched regularly, the greater her risk. After fifteen years of regularly douching, the risk of an ectopic pregnancy was seven to eight and a half times that of a woman who had never douched. An estimated 37 percent of American women douche; if you are among them, discontinue the practice, at least until you have finished having children.

Take Cough Syrup

Guaifenesin, the active ingredient in Robitussin and several other cough syrups, works by thinning the mucus in the lungs. As an added benefit, it also thins the cervical mucus, making it better suited for moving sperm through the reproductive organs. Take one to two teaspoons a day, starting three or four days before ovulation.

HIS

Ejaculate Every Two or Three Days

You're going to have to pace yourself: Ejaculating too much—or too little—can lower your sperm count. Don't believe the old wives' tale about "storing up" sperm to promote conception.

Most infertile couples focus on the timing of intercourse near the anticipated time of ovulation, but it is helpful to enjoy your sex life all month long. While absence may make the heart grow fonder, studies have found that abstinence makes the sperm grow weaker. Researchers have found that waiting more than two or three days between ejaculations (whether through intercourse or masturbation) can lead to a diminished number of active sperm and inferior sperm quality. Regular sexual activity increases testosterone levels, which stimulates sperm production and maturation. So to maximize your sperm count, enjoy a rewarding sex life all month long, not just around the time of ovulation.

Take a Cold Bath—Before Sex, Not Instead of It

"Go take a cold shower" may be one way of turning down the heat when someone's amorous ambitions cannot be acted on, but evidence suggests that a cold bath or shower thirty minutes before intercourse can actually improve fertility. Evidence indicates that a cold bath increases the flow of oxygen in the body and the level of testosterone in the blood. So you might as well try a five-minute soak to cool things off—then enjoy yourself as things heat up.

Consult a Doctor if You Have Very Little Seminal Fluid

In some cases, a physical problem can cause a man to ejaculate into his bladder, rather than out through the end of the penis. He enjoys the pleasurable sensations associated with an orgasm, but no fluid is released. Then, the next time he urinates, a milky white fluid—semen—is excreted along with the urine.

In many cases, this problem, known as retrograde ejaculation, stems from a neurological disorder that causes a lack of control of the muscles at the base of the bladder that normally close off just before ejaculation. (The nerve damage can be a complication of diabetes.) Retrograde ejaculation can also be a side effect of certain medications, including those used to treat depression and hypertension. A change in medications or, in some cases, surgery can be effective in treating the problem.

Keep in mind that the volume of ejaculate is not a reflection of the number of sperm a man is producing. A man can be sterile and produce a tablespoon of semen, while potent men can release just a drop or two. As for average, most men release between one-half and one teaspoon of ejaculate.

A SEASON FOR LOVE

If your sperm count is low, check the calendar. According to researchers at the University of Texas Health Center in Houston, sperm counts fluctuate throughout the year, peaking between February and March, and falling to the lowest levels in September. No wonder Valentine's Day is February 14.

Treat Impotence

Don't be embarrassed: Sooner or later, most men experience occasional episodes of impotence. However, an ongoing problem with impotence—the inability to achieve and maintain a successful erection—can obviously interfere with fertility. Fortunately, impotence and problems of sexual dysfunction affect only about 5 percent of infertile men.

Many erection problems have at least some physical cause. To achieve an erection there must be cooperation of blood vessels, nerves, and tissues. Impotence can be caused by a number of health problems, including diabetes, heart and circulation problems, stroke, epilepsy, Alzheimer's disease, neurological disorders, alcohol and drug abuse, Parkinson's disease, and liver and kidney disease. Impotence can also be caused by certain medications, such as tranquilizers, diuretics, and anti-ulcer, anti-psychotic, anti-depressant, and anti-hypertensive drugs. Some over-the-counter antihistamines and decongestants can cause temporary impotence as well.

The other cases of impotence stem from psychological factors, such as relationship problems, stress, anxiety, grief, depression, fatigue, boredom, and guilt. Sexual intimacy can make some people feel very vulnerable, causing a number of stresses and uncomfortable feelings.

With patience and treatment, most cases of impotence can be managed and overcome, but you must be willing to ask for help. The prescription drug Viagra, approved by the FDA last year, has been shown to help 70 percent of men with impotence. For more information on impotence, talk to your doctor or contact:

Potency Restored
8630 Fenton Street, Suite 218
Silver Spring, MD 20910
(301) 588-5777

Impotence Institute of America
10400 Little Patuxent Parkway, Suite 485
Columbia, MD 21044
(410) 715-9605

Impotence Information Center
American Medical Systems
Minneapolis, MN 55440
(800) 543-9632

COUPLES

Be Conventional: Stick to the Missionary Position

The so-called missionary sexual position—man on top, woman on the bottom—reduces the risk of sperm leaking from the vagina and increases contact of the semen with the cervix. If you are a woman, after intercourse you might want to tip your hips back, slip a pillow or two under your hips, and gently press the labia (lips) of your vagina together to give the sperm every chance possible to work their way north to the Fallopian tubes.

Another option is rear entry or "doggie style." This position allows for the deposit of sperm close to the cervix. When you're trying to conceive, don't make love sitting, standing, or with the woman on top.

Make Love Before You Make Breakfast

Making love is a nice way to say good morning. There are no studies to show that morning intercourse improves the odds of conception, but experts do know that sperm counts are higher in the morning (provided you haven't had intercourse the night before). In addition, male hormones peak in the morning, which may help explain why many men feel passionate first thing in the morning.

Have Sex Every Other Day

Some infertile couples assume that conception can most easily be achieved by having intercourse as often as possible near the time of ovulation. However, too much of a good thing can compromise sperm count.

Your goal, of course, is to fertilize a mature egg as soon as possible after it is released from the ovary. Since this window of opportunity can be just six or eight hours for some women, intercourse must occur in a timely fashion. Mother Nature makes this task somewhat easier because sperm can survive inside the vagina for up to five days. (Actually, the length of time the sperm remain alive depends on where a woman is in her menstrual cycle: If she is in an infertile phase, the sperm will die within hours; if she is approaching ovulation, the sperm can survive for days in the more hospitable wet cervical mucus.)

Waiting two days between lovemaking sessions is ideal for most couples. Having intercourse daily will reduce sperm count somewhat, which can make a difference in cases where the man has low or borderline sperm count. One exception: Men who have excessively high sperm counts (as determined by a sperm analysis conducted by a doctor) may find that daily intercourse helps lower the sperm count to a more normal level, which can prevent the sperm from fighting one another.

Don't try to "save up" sperm by avoiding intercourse for a week or more before ovulation. This period of abstinence will lower sperm production, and it will result in the release of a large number of old sperm cells, which are less likely to achieve fertilization.

Also, keep in mind that the slippery, clear fluid or gel that is released prior to ejaculation contains live sperm. This pre-ejaculate is designed to protect the sperm by neutralizing acids in the urethra and vagina. Don't confuse the release of this fluid with premature ejaculation; when ejaculation occurs, the prostate will release a greater supply of fluid that will allow the sperm to travel in the vaginal canal.

Choosing the Sex of Your Baby

If you're having trouble getting pregnant, you probably don't care about the sex of your child—you just want to have a healthy baby. But, to the degree that you can choose, some people like to try to tip the scales in favor of one sex or the other.

It's the sperm that determine the sex of the baby. The male sperm (with Y chromosomes) tend to be smaller, lighter, faster, and more fragile than the female sperm (with X chromosomes), which tend to be bigger, heavier, slower, and longer-lived. While these methods are far from foolproof, evidence does suggest that the timing of intercourse can influence the sex of the baby. Consider the fact that fraternal twins (which come from two separate eggs) tend to be the same sex, and they would have been fertilized at the same time.

FOR A GIRL

- Make love using shallow penetration in the missionary position; this will deposit the sperm at the mouth of the cervix and favor the slower-swimming female sperm.
- The woman should avoid orgasm; this will keep the vaginal canal relatively acidic, which will tend to kill off male sperm in favor of female sperm.
- Make love on the second or third day before you anticipate ovulation. This will allow the longer-lasting female sperm to be present in the Fallopian tube at the time the egg is released from the ovary.

FOR A BOY

- Make love using deep penetration (perhaps in the rear-entry position), which will deposit the sperm at the neck of the cervix, where they can sprint inside the uterus and speed their way up to the Fallopian tubes. In addition, the area deep inside the vagina tends to be more alkaline and more hospitable to male sperm.
- The woman should have an orgasm; this will create a more male-sperm-friendly alkaline environment.
- Make love as close to the time of ovulation as possible; this will allow the energetic, fast-swimming male sperm to reach the egg first. Also have intercourse on the day following your perceived peak day, just in case you miscalculated.

Skip Oral Sex

The bacteria found in saliva can degrade semen and reduce the chances of conception. Studies have found that saliva significantly decreases sperm motility and progression, causing many sperm to shake and vibrate without moving forward. Both partners should avoid giving or receiving oral sex during those lovemaking sessions in which you are trying to get pregnant.

Don't Have Intercourse Under Water

While making love in a pool or on the beach can be erotic and exciting, under-water intercourse can undermine your chances of conceiving a child. The chlorine found in the pool water can alter the vaginal pH level, and the presence of any water can wash away or alter the all-important vaginal mucus, which helps the sperm work its way to the awaiting egg.

Avoid Commercial Vaginal Lubricants

Massage oils and lubricating jellies, liquids, and suppositories may enhance lovemaking, but they may inhibit babymaking at the same time. Many commercial lubricants can interfere with the sperm's ability to make its way through the reproductive tract. Oil-based lubricants, such as petroleum jelly, can alter the vaginal pH and damage sperm. Even water-based products (usually marked "safe to use with condoms") can slow down or trap sperm.

Instead of using commercial products, use egg white if you really need a lubricant. The egg white is pure protein—and so are the sperm—and the egg white won't disrupt the natural pH balance in the vagina.

Note: Do not use egg white if either partner is allergic to eggs. Be sure to separate the yolk from the egg before using egg white as a lubricant.

Consider Whether Either Partner Has Anti-sperm Antibodies

Anti-sperm antibodies are evidence of an overzealous immune system. When the immune system is working as it should, the white blood cells produce proteins known as antibodies, which seek out and destroy hostile proteins, known as antigens. These antigens attack a range of foreign invaders—viruses, bacteria, fungi, and other microorganisms that can cause illness. Sometimes, however, the body mistakenly sets its sights on harmless proteins, such as sperm. When antibodies attach themselves to the sperm, they can cause problems with motility and the ability of the sperm to penetrate the egg.

Experts disagree about how often anti-sperm antibodies cause infertility, but some believe the condition exists in up to 20 percent of infertile women and 10 percent of infertile men. Many researchers believe that the antibodies can reduce the chances of conception, but do not necessarily prevent it.

In women, experts believe the problem can be triggered by infection, though the condition is not very well understood. In men, anti-sperm antibodies sometimes appear after vasectomy; the condition can also follow infection or injury to the genital area. Lab tests involving blood, cervical mucus, and sperm will be needed to detect the presence of the antibodies.

If a man has anti-sperm antibodies, he should work

with a urologist with expertise in fertility to take steps to manage the problem. If a woman has developed antibodies to her partner's sperm, the problem can be corrected in some cases by having the man wear a condom during intercourse and oral sex for six months to give the woman's immune system a chance to stop forming antibodies. Then, after this period of rest, it is possible that the couple can have intercourse without a condom at the time of ovulation and pregnancy can occur before the antibodies form again. If you have this problem, this low-tech approach is certainly worth a try, and some researchers have reported success rates of up to 50 percent using this technique. If this method does not work, do not despair. Many couples with immunological disorders can conceive with the help of assisted reproductive technologies.

This is a complex problem that will probably require diagnosis and treatment from a physician. If either partner has a history of infections or sexually transmitted diseases, consult a fertility expert to find out if anti-sperm antibodies are contributing to your problems with conception. Keep in mind that the low-tech techniques described in this book cannot help you if anti-sperm antibodies are present.

Test for Sexually Transmitted Diseases and Treat Them Promptly

Sexually transmitted diseases (STDs) can scar the reproductive system and cause infertility in both women and men. Americans report 12 million new cases of STDs and 1 million cases of pelvic inflammatory disease each year, according to the Centers for Disease Control and Prevention in Atlanta. About 12.5 percent of these infections lead to infertility after a single episode, and an astonishing 75 percent of people are left infertile after three infections. (People who smoke are particularly susceptible to scarring and infertility because smoking slows down the healing process.)

In women, pelvic inflammatory disease (PID) is almost always sexually transmitted. It can be caused by any of a number of organisms, but once they reach the vagina during intercourse, they spread throughout the reproductive system. PID is often found in women who have had multiple sex partners, especially in couples who did not use a barrier form of contraception (such as condoms or diaphragms). It can also be caused by abortion and the use of IUDs (intrauterine devices). PID may show up as pelvic pain, odorous vaginal discharge, vaginal bleeding, painful urination, fever, chills, nausea, and vomiting—or it can be present without any symptoms at all. Ideally, a woman should have a complete gynecological exam before trying to conceive, so that her doctor can identify and treat any harmful microorganisms that might be present.

In men, the sperm are produced in the testicles, then they must move along an eighteen-foot, tightly coiled tube known as the epididymis. The sperm must then travel through the vas deferens, the tube connecting the epididymis and the prostate gland. Many sexually transmitted diseases can cause tubular scarring and infertility; blocked sperm ducts account for an estimated 10 to 15 percent of male infertility. The more sex partners a man has had, the greater the number and type of bacteria he will have in his prostate gland and seminal fluid, and the greater the chance that these bacteria will cause PID in his female partners.

For both women and men, the best way to protect your fertility and to minimize your risk of developing STDs is to limit your number of sexual partners, use condoms, and seek medical care as soon as symptoms appear. In many cases, the damage caused by an STD is irreversible—and the damage is done before the infection is diagnosed and treated. For more information on sexually transmitted diseases, contact your gynecologist or another physician.

FERTILITY CHECKLIST

HERS

- ❑ Calculate your anticipated day of ovulation using the calendar method.
- ❑ Learn to recognize changes in your cervical mucus.
- ❑ Chart the changes in your basal body temperature.
- ❑ Monitor changes in your cervix.
- ❑ Try an ovulation predictor kit.
- ❑ Stay flat on your back for 20 to 30 minutes after intercourse.
- ❑ Don't douche.
- ❑ Take a cough syrup with guaifenesin.

HIS

- ❑ Ejaculate every two or three days all month.
- ❑ Take a cold bath a half-hour before sex.
- ❑ Talk to your doctor if you release little or no seminal fluid at orgasm.
- ❑ Treat impotence.

COUPLES

- ❑ Use the missionary position.
- ❑ Make love in the morning.
- ❑ Have intercourse every other day.
- ❑ Avoid oral sex.
- ❑ Don't have intercourse under water.
- ❑ Avoid pharmaceutical vaginal lubricants.
- ❑ Consider whether either partner has anti-sperm antibodies.
- ❑ Test for sexually transmitted diseases and treat them promptly.

3

Nutrition and Nutrition Supplements: Eat, Drink — and Get Pregnant

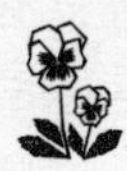

If you're thinking about getting pregnant, you need to begin eating for two *before* you conceive. You don't necessarily need to eat more, but you may need to eat better. Eating a balanced diet high in certain nutrients can help to improve your fertility. And changing your diet is easier—and much less expensive and potentially harmful—than experimenting with reproductive technologies.

But it's often difficult, even under the best of circumstances, to get all the vitamins and minerals you need for optimal fertility from the foods you eat. The best way to make up for the shortcomings in your diet and to be sure you meet your minimum nutritional requirements is to take daily prenatal multivitamins at least six months before you want to conceive. In addition, other nutrition supplements can be used to enhance your fertility.

Shopping for Supplements

- When shopping for nutrition supplements, look for store brands. All vitamins and nutrition supplements are essentially the same, so skip the brand-name products and look for the bargains. If you reach only for the heavily advertised brands, all you're doing is helping the manufacturer pay for its advertising.
- Don't pay more for "natural" vitamins and supplements. The biggest difference between natural and synthetic vitamins is cost. Nutrition supplements that come from the laboratory are chemically identical to those that come from the farm. One important exception is vitamin E. The body can absorb and use natural vitamin E more easily than the synthetic version.
- Check the expiration date on the bottle before you buy. Nutrition supplements lose potency over time. The bottle should bear a "freshness and potency guaranteed through" date somewhere on the label.

HERS

Take Up to 10,000 IU of Vitamin A Daily as Part of a Multivitamin Supplement

Vitamin A is important in the function of the reproductive glands, which regulate ovulation and influence sexual energy. In fact, fish liver oil—a rich source of vitamin A—is a time-honored remedy among Native Americans for women who experience difficulty conceiving. Vitamin A also assists in the metabolism of fat and helps with the healthy function of the eyes, hair, teeth, gums, and mucous membranes.

Vitamin A in animal tissues is called retinol; vitamin A in plants is called beta-carotene. (Beta-carotene is sometimes called a provitamin because it must be broken down by the body into vitamin A before it acts as a vitamin.) Both vitamin A and beta-carotene are antioxidants; they help protect the body from cancer and improve resistance to certain diseases by neutralizing damaging free radicals.

Vitamin A and beta-carotene should not be taken in large amounts—more than 10,000 IU (international units)—in pill form or as cod liver oil by pregnant women, diabetics, and people with hypothyroidism or liver disease. (Excessive vitamin A during pregnancy can cause birth defects.) Antibiotics, laxatives, and some cholesterol-lowering drugs can interfere with the body's ability to absorb vitamin A. Signs of vitamin A deficiency include night blindness, retarded growth, impaired resistance to disease, infection, rough skin, and dry eyes. About 15 percent of all Americans are deficient in vitamin A.

Good Food Sources of Vitamin A

- Fish oils
- Dairy products: whole milk, cream, butter, fortified margarine, eggs, cheese
- Green leafy vegetables
- Yellow and orange vegetables and fruits
- Organ meats
- Red peppers

Take Up to 50 Milligrams of Vitamin B6 Three Times a Day as Part of a B-complex Supplement

Vitamin B6 (pyridoxine) is essential for the function of the reproductive glands. It also assists in the metabolism of proteins, carbohydrates, and fats; aids the formation of red blood cells; and helps in the functioning of the nervous system and brain. It is also required by at least fifty different enzymes in various metabolic processes throughout the body.

Studies have shown that vitamin B6 significantly increases progesterone levels and improves fertility. In one study of fourteen women with unexplained infertility, twelve became pregnant after taking high doses of vitamin B6 (100 to 800 milligrams daily) for six months. The women ranged in age from twenty-three to thirty-one; they had been infertile from eighteen months to seven years.

Do not take more than 150 milligrams of vitamin B6 a day without consulting a doctor. Megadoses of vitamin B6 can cause peripheral nerve damage. High doses of one B vitamin can also throw the others out of balance, since they tend to work together in the body.

Signs of vitamin B6 deficiency include depression, confusion, convulsions, irritability, insomnia, reduced resistance to infection, sores in the mouth, and itchy skin. Be aware that taking antidepressants, supplemental estrogen, and oral contraceptives may increase the need for vitamin B6. Women who have taken birth control pills tend to experience vitamin B6 deficiency more often than those who have not.

Take Up to 2.5 Milligrams of Copper Daily

Copper is necessary for the maintenance of healthy blood cells and bones. Studies have found that infertile women have significantly lower concentrations of copper

Good Food Sources of Vitamin B6

* Meats and poultry
* Grains: whole-grain cereals, wheat germ
* Brewer's yeast
* Fish
* Eggs
* Carrots
* Nuts: hazelnuts, cashews, peanuts, walnuts
* Sunflower seeds
* Lentils and legumes
* Rice
* Avocados
* Bananas

in their blood plasma than fertile women do. Signs of copper deficiency include anemia and elevated blood cholesterol levels. Be aware that high levels of zinc and vitamin C can reduce copper levels.

Take Up to 500 Milligrams of Evening Primrose Oil Three Times a Day

The oil from the seeds of the evening primrose plant contains gamma-linolenic acid, an oil much like the essential fatty acid omega-6. A deficiency in the essential

GOOD FOOD SOURCES OF COPPER

- Shellfish
- Organ meats: liver, kidney
- Fish
- Nuts
- Legumes
- Mushrooms
- Molasses and honey
- Wheat germ and whole-grain cereals

fatty acids can contribute to infertility by causing a thickening of the cervical mucus and the formation of mucus hostile to sperm. Evening primrose oil—as well as fish oils—contains fatty acids that can help reverse infertility caused by a mucus problem.

The gamma-linolenic acid found in evening primrose oil is also a precursor to the formation of certain prostaglandins, which help reduce inflammation, lower blood pressure, maintain salt-water balance, and support the immune system. While side effects from evening primrose oil are quite rare, you can avoid nausea by taking the supplements with food.

GOOD SOURCES OF EVENING PRIMROSE OIL

- Evening primrose oil is commercially available as a nutrition supplement. Look for a product that contains 35 to 40 milligrams of GLA—gamma-linolenic acid—per 500 milligram capsule.

HIS

Take Up to 4 Grams of Arginine Daily

Arginine is considered a "nonessential" amino acid, but it may be essential to the formation of healthy sperm. This makes sense when you consider that arginine is required for the replication of cells, including the formation of sperm cells.

Studies have shown that taking 4 grams of powdered arginine dissolved in water can significantly boost sperm counts and sperm motility in some men, especially those with only moderately depressed sperm counts. One study of 178 men found significant improvement in sperm count and sperm motility in almost three out of four men included in the study who took 4 grams of arginine a day.

It may take several months for results, so try to be patient. You should take amino acids on an empty stomach for optimal absorption. They can be purchased as capsules, tablets, and powders, either alone, as protein mixtures, or in multivitamin formulas.

GOOD FOOD SOURCES OF ARGININE

* Animal protein
* Brown rice
* Eggs
* Milk
* Yeast

Avoid Consuming Any Cottonseed Oil

While you may not think of foods as contraceptives, cottonseed oil is a rich source of gossypol, an anti-fertility agent that has been examined as a possible active ingredient for a "male birth control pill." Studies have actually shown that men who use crude cottonseed oil in cooking have low sperm counts and testicular problems. Read your food labels carefully and avoid any product containing cottonseed oil. It is most commonly used in fried foods. (Of course, you cannot rely on cottonseed oil to prevent pregnancy when you want to use a contraceptive, but you should by all means avoid it when you're trying to get pregnant.)

Take Up to 500 Milligrams of L-carnitine Daily

L-carnitine is a vitaminlike compound that stimulates energy-producing mitochondria in the cells to break down long-chain fatty acids. L-carnitine levels run quite high in the epididymis (the tube in the scrotum where the sperm are formed) and in the sperm themselves. L-carnitine levels in the body have a direct relationship to sperm vitality: the higher the L-carnitine concentration, the more motile the sperm. L-carnitine is found in the diet and can also be produced by the body, mainly in the liver and kidneys.

Taking a L-carnitine supplement can help boost fertility. Look for a product labeled L-carnitine, rather than D-carnitine or DL-carnitine. (The L-carnitine is in a molecular form that is more easily used by the body; in some people, the D-form actually creates an L-carnitine defi-

GOOD FOOD SOURCES OF CARNITINE

- Red meats
- Fish
- Poultry
- Milk and dairy products
- Whole wheat
- Avocados

ciency.) Supplemental L-carnitine is not recommended for diabetics or people with liver or kidney disease.

Take Up to 200 Micrograms of Selenium Daily

Fertile men need selenium; it is necessary for healthy sperm production and for a healthy sex drive. It is also critical for liver, heart, and white blood cell function, and it contributes to the breakdown of fat in the body.

While researchers don't fully understand the role of selenium and fertility, they do know that almost half of a male's selenium supply can be found in the testicles and the seminal ducts next to the prostate gland. Since selenium is a powerful antioxidant, it may work by protecting the sperm from the hazards of exposure to damaging free radicals. Men with low levels of selenium—and consequently high levels of exposure to free radicals—are much more likely to have abnormal sperm and low sperm counts, compared to men who are not exposed to free radical damage. In fact, high levels of free radicals are found in the semen of 40 percent of infertile men.

Signs of selenium deficiency include liver disease, skin problems, and arthritis.

GOOD FOOD SOURCES OF SELENIUM

Note: The selenium content of foods is highly variable because of the wide variability of this element in the soil.

- Fish and shellfish
- Organ meats
- Whole grains
- Brewer's yeast
- Dairy products, especially egg yolks
- Molasses
- Mushrooms
- Brazil nuts

Eat a Diet Rich in Soy Foods

To boost your testosterone level and promote fertility, have a heaping helping of legumes, seeds, or other soy-rich foods. Soy is a good source of isoflavonoids or phytoestrogens, compounds that function like a mild form of estrogen in the body. These compounds actually bind to estrogen receptors, preventing the body's own estrogen from binding to the receptor. Making a few changes in your diet may be enough to help if your testosterone levels are marginal or low.

Good Food Sources of Soy

- Soybeans
- Soy flour
- Soy milk
- Textured soy protein
- Tofu
- Miso
- Tempeh
- Legumes
- Nuts and seeds

Four Simple Ways to Add Soy to Your Diet

1. In baking, substitute one-third cup of soy flour and two-thirds cup of wheat flour per cup of flour in recipes.
2. Use soy milk instead of cow's milk.
3. Use textured vegetable protein instead of ground beef in recipes.
4. Snack on roasted soy nuts.

Take Up to 10 Micrograms of Vitamin B12 Daily as Part of a B-complex Supplement

Vitamin B12 is involved in cellular replication and the

Good Food Sources of Vitamin B12

- Organ meats: liver, kidney
- Dairy products: milk, eggs, yogurt, cheese (especially Camembert and Gorgonzola)
- Fish and shellfish
- Meat: beef, poultry, pork

formation of genetic material and red blood cells. A deficiency of vitamin B12 (or cyanocobalamine) can lead to reduced sperm count and sperm motility. Even in the absence of a vitamin B12 deficiency, taking supplements seems to stoke the body's sperm manufacturing systems. In one study, men with low sperm counts (less than 20 million per milliliter) took 1,000 micrograms of vitamin B12 daily. By the end of the study, almost one out of three men had achieved a total sperm count of more than 100 million. You should not take megadoses of vitamin B12 without consulting a doctor; high levels of one B vitamin can cause an imbalance in the other B vitamins. However, taking a moderate dose as part of a B-complex supplement may help overcome a vitamin deficiency that may be contributing to your infertility problems.

Be aware that anti-gout medications, anticoagulant drugs, and potassium supplements may block the absorption of vitamin B12, possibly contributing to a vitamin deficiency.

Take Up to 3,000 Milligrams of Vitamin C Daily

Vitamin C (ascorbic acid) can almost be considered a wonder vitamin, especially when it comes to fertility. In the body, it helps bind cells together and strengthens the walls of the blood vessels; it helps fight infection; it promotes wound healing—and it does a fabulous job of promoting healthy sperm. Vitamin C levels are much higher in seminal fluid compared to other body fluids, including the blood.

Studies have shown that men who took as little as 1,000 milligrams of vitamin C daily showed increased sperm count and improved sperm motility and longevity. One study looked at the impact of vitamin C deficiency on sperm clumping, a problem that contributes to infertility because sperm must swim alone in order to build enough momentum to penetrate and fertilize an egg. (The experts say that a clumped sperm figure of more than 25 percent often separates fertile from infertile men.) Researchers looked at thirty-five young men with high rates of sperm clumping; they found that all the men had low levels of vitamin C in their blood. But vitamin C offered a simple and effective cure: After just one week with a daily supplement of 1 gram of vitamin C, the men had normal levels of vitamin C in their blood and normal sperm motility.

Researchers at the University of California at Berkeley have found that vitamin C also helps protect sperm's genetic material—its DNA—from damage caused by free radicals in the body. To test the role of vitamin C on sperm, the researchers at Berkeley reduced the dietary vitamin C intake in healthy male subjects from 250 milligrams to just 5 milligrams per day. In response to this vitamin C deficiency, the vitamin C levels in the seminal fluid dropped by 50 percent and the number of sperm with damaged DNA shot up by 91 percent. When the men resumed their normal diet (which included 60 to 250 milligrams of vitamin C), the DNA damage to the sperm declined within one month. The bottom line: Vitamin C not only helps prevent infertility, it may also help prevent birth defects in offspring.

Be aware that the use of aspirin, alcohol, analgesics, antidepressants, anticoagulants, and steroids may reduce vitamin C levels in the body. Medications for diabetes and sulfa drugs may not be as effective when taken with vitamin C. Signs of vitamin C deficiency include scurvy, bleeding gums, loose teeth, slow healing, dry and rough skin, and loss of appetite.

GOOD FOOD SOURCES OF VITAMIN C

- Rose hips
- Fruits: oranges, pineapples, grapefruit, lemon, lime, kiwi, mangos, cantaloupe, cherries, papayas, strawberries, tomatoes
- Peppers (red, yellow, and green)
- Green vegetables, especially broccoli, Brussels sprouts, and spinach
- Avocados
- Cauliflower
- New potatoes
- Onions
- Radishes
- Watercress
- Calves' liver

COUPLES

Take Up to 800 IU of Vitamin E Daily

Vitamin E is necessary for balanced hormone production in both women and men. It also helps the body form red blood cells, muscles, and other tissues, and it is necessary for the breakdown of fats.

Vitamin E has been shown to improve sperm count and motility. In the laboratory, it has been found to enhance the ability of sperm to fertilize eggs in test tubes. As an antioxidant, it also helps protect cell membranes—including sperm membranes—from free radical damage.

The body needs zinc to maintain the proper levels of vitamin E in the blood, so you might consider taking supplemental zinc as well as vitamin E. People suffering from diabetes, heart disease, or thyroid disorders should not use this vitamin without consulting a physician.

GOOD FOOD SOURCES OF VITAMIN E

Note: Vitamin E is the only vitamin destroyed by freezing; it is also nutritionally diminished by exposure to extreme heat.

- Wheat germ
- Whole-grain cereals and breads
- Green vegetables
- Nuts: almonds, Brazil nuts, cashews, hazelnuts, peanuts, walnuts
- Vegetable oils

Take Up to 50 Milligrams of Zinc Daily

Zinc is an essential mineral for both female and male reproductive health. In women, zinc deficiency can lead to hormone imbalance, abnormal ovarian development, and menstrual irregularity. Once a woman is pregnant, zinc deficiency can also increase the risk of miscarriage, stillbirth, pregnancy-related high blood pressure, and low-birth-weight infants.

In men, zinc is important for the healthy functioning of the prostate gland and the reproductive organs. This mineral is crucial for cell division, growth, and repair, and it plays a role in the metabolism of carbohydrates and vitamins. Low levels of zinc can cause a loss of taste, delayed wound healing, and infertility.

Even mild zinc deficiency can lead to low sperm count. Fortunately, taking supplemental zinc can improve sperm count and motility. One study of thirty-seven infertile men involved the use of 60 milligrams of

Good Food Sources of Zinc

- Meat, poultry, pork
- Eggs
- Seafood, especially oysters and herring
- Whole grains and wheat germ
- Brewer's yeast
- Seeds: sesame seeds, sunflower seeds, pumpkin seeds
- Bonemeal
- Molasses and maple syrup

zinc sulfate for forty to fifty days. Of the men with low testosterone levels, sperm counts increased by 8 million to 20 million. Other studies have demonstrated an improvement in semen quality and motility.

Zinc also appears to play a role in regulating sex drive, adding credibility to the use of oysters as a male aphrodisiac. (Just six medium eastern oysters contain a whopping 76 milligrams of zinc.)

FERTILITY CHECKLIST

HERS

- ❑ Vitamin A: up to 10,000 IU daily.
- ❑ Vitamin B6: up to 50 milligrams three times a day.
- ❑ Copper: up to 2.5 milligrams daily.
- ❑ Evening primrose oil: up to 500 milligrams three times a day.

HIS

- ❑ Arginine: up to 4 grams daily.
- ❑ Cottonseed oil: Avoid.
- ❑ L-carnitine: up to 500 milligrams daily.
- ❑ Selenium: up to 200 micrograms daily.
- ❑ Soy: eat a diet rich in soy foods.
- ❑ Vitamin B12: up to 10 micrograms daily.
- ❑ Vitamin C: up to 3,000 milligrams daily.

COUPLES

- ❑ Vitamin E: up to 800 IU daily.
- ❑ Zinc: up to 50 milligrams daily.

4

Herbs: Mother Nature's Medicines for Maternity

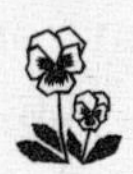

Getting pregnant is a balancing act. For both women and men, fertility involves a complex hormonal chain reaction; for the system to work, the entire system has to be in working order.

All too often, low levels of a hormone may knock the system out of balance, inhibiting fertility. While synthetic drugs like clomid or perganol can stimulate egg release, sometimes more subtle treatments—such as herbal remedies—can jump start the hormonal system, often without the undesirable side effects of the stronger drugs.

Every culture on earth has relied on the natural healing ability of plants (or botanicals) to treat many ailments. Worldwide, four out of five people use herbs as the basis of their medical care. Though most Americans rely on synthetic drugs produced in a laboratory, European doctors often prescribe herbal treatments for their patients. One of the main reasons that synthetic medicines are more popular than herbs in the United States is that drug companies can patent those drugs they create, but they cannot patent Mother Nature's cures. Still, about 25 percent of all prescription drugs sold in the United States contain active ingredients isolated from plants, and most synthetic drugs are little more than synthesized versions of chemicals that occur naturally in plants.

STRONG MEDICINE

Many people who agonize over taking an over-the-counter painkiller think nothing of swallowing an herbal treatment because they consider it "natural" and therefore not dangerous. But herbs powerful enough to heal are also powerful enough to harm, if misused. In general, herbal remedies are safer and have fewer side effects than man-made drugs, but they can be as potent and as harmful as synthetic drugs, and they should be treated with the same respect. Like any other drugs, herbs can have negative and sometimes dangerous side effects if taken in excessive doses. When it comes to herbs—as with many things—more is not necessarily better.

Part of the confusion about safety stems from the way

herbal treatments are labeled. Unlike synthetic drugs, herbal remedies do not have to go through the formal approval process from the U.S. Food and Drug Administration because they are classified as foods or food additives, rather than drugs. This means that manufacturers of herbal remedies must be cautious about the claims they make on package labels; drug-related claims and warnings are prohibited. It's up to you to understand the safety and efficacy of the products you buy. You should always read the package directions and follow the dosage information on the product label. If you have any questions about how a product should be used, contact the manufacturer for more information.

You can find many herbal remedies in health food stores, but in recent years they have been showing up in conventional supermarkets and pharmacies as well. If you can't find what you need at local stores, refer to the listing on pages 183-184 for information on mail-order companies that sell herbs.

USING HERBS

While all herbal medicines rely on plant materials, different medicines use different parts of the plant, such as the leaves, seeds, flowers, roots, bark, or berries. The particular "recipes" for herbal remedies have been refined and improved by herbalists over thousands of years. Though only a tiny fraction of the world's plants have been tested for their medicinal potential, American herbalists use more than one thousand different herbs to treat a wide range of illnesses and medical conditions. The following remedies are among the key treatments for infertility.

Regardless of what plants they are made of, herbal medicines come in one of several forms, including:

* **Teas:** Made by steeping one teaspoon of dried herbs or three teaspoons of fresh herbs in one cup of boiling water for five minutes or so, then straining. Most herbal teas are not strong enough to provide medicinal value, so in most cases you can drink as much herbal tea as you wish.
* **Infusions:** Made much the same way as strong tea, with several important exceptions. The water should be just short of boiling (since boiling water releases important volatile oils in the steam), and the herbs are steeped for twenty to thirty minutes, so the resulting liquid is much more potent and often more bitter than tea. The infusion should be strained before drinking. Most infusions are made with one-half to one rounded teaspoon of dried herb or three teaspoons of fresh herb per cup

of water. The standard dose for most infusions is one-half cup, three times a day.

✸ **Decoctions:** Made like infusions, only the bark, roots, or berries of the herbs are simmered (never boiled), rather than merely steeped, for twenty to thirty minutes (or sometimes longer). Most decoctions are made with one-half to one rounded teaspoon of dried herb per cup of water. The standard dose for most decoctions is one-half cup, three times a day.

✸ **Tinctures:** Made by soaking herbs in an alcohol solution (25 percent alcohol/75 percent water) for a specified period of time (from several hours to several days, depending on the herb). Commercial tinctures use ethyl alcohol, but apple cider vinegar, vodka, brandy, and rum are suitable for home use (and the brandy and rum can help to disguise the bitter flavor of some herbs). Because alcohol acts as a preservative, tinctures can be stored for up to two years. To prepare a tincture, soak one ounce of crushed dried herbs in five ounces of distilled spirits for six weeks. Shake the mixture every few days to encourage alcohol uptake of the herb's active ingredients. The dosage for a tincture depends on the herb being used. *Warning:* Do not use methyl alcohol or isopropyl alcohol (rubbing alcohol) when making tinctures; they are toxic if taken internally.

✸ **Extracts:** Made by distilling some of the alcohol off

a tincture, leaving a more potent concentrate behind. Most commercial extracts use vacuum distillation or filtration techniques, which do not require the use of high temperatures. The dosage for an extract depends on the herb being used.

✸ **Powdered herbs:** Made by removing the moisture from an extract, then grinding the solid herbal concentrate into granules or powders, which can be shaped into capsules or tablets. The dosage for powdered herbs depends on the herb being used.

Most of the herbal treatments mentioned in this book involve infusions or decoctions, which may have a sharp, bitter taste. If you don't care for the flavor of an herbal remedy, try covering the unpleasant flavor with sugar, honey, lemon, fruit juice, or even flavored tea mix. You can also purchase prepared tinctures, extracts, or powdered herbs and follow the dosage information on the product labels.

Before using herbs, check with your doctor, since herbal medicines can interact with some conventional drugs. Use only the recommended amounts and take herbs only for the recommended time periods. The risk of side effects goes up when people take large amounts of herbs for extended periods. Start with a low-strength preparation and strengthen it only if necessary.

Watch out for symptoms of overdose or toxicity. Typical symptoms include stomach upset, nausea, diarrhea, or headache an hour or two after taking an herb. If you develop any suspicious symptoms after taking an herb, stop taking it and see if the symptoms disappear. If you have an adverse reaction, report it to the U.S. Food and Drug Administration's MedWatch office at (800) 332-1088.

—— Q & A ——

Which herbs should I take?

All the herbs discussed in this chapter can help to enhance your fertility. However, different herbs address different fertility problems, so be sure to read the description of each herb carefully to see if it will help with your particular problem.

Most of the herbal treatments listed in this book involve single herbs, rather than formulas, or blends of herbs designed to act synergistically to achieve specific results for a specific individual. If you plan to experiment with herbal remedies on your own, try one or two of the herbs suggested in this chapter. If you are interested in a multiherb fertility formula, look in your local health food store, or consult a professional herbalist who can prepare a blend designed to meet your individual needs.

How much should I take?

Most of the remedies discussed in this chapter involve infusions made with loose herbs. The dosage is listed with the information on each herb. Some people prefer to use commercially prepared products. Of course, follow all package directions for dosage information.

Are the herbs listed here safe?

As mentioned earlier, herbs generally have fewer side effects than synthetic drugs, but they can be dangerous if misused. For each herb discussed in this chapter, there is a list of precautions, which describes who should not use a particular herb and what the possible side effects might be. Keep in mind, however, that the side effects tend to appear only at doses in excess of the amounts recommended here.

HERS

Black Cohosh *(Cimicifuga racemosa)*

This herb is estrogen-promoting and anti-spasmodic. In fact, one of the nineteenth century's most popular patent medicines contained black cohosh and was used to treat "female weakness" or menstrual cramps. The herb was used for centuries by the Algonquian Indians in the treatment of gynecological problems.

Usage: For a decoction, simmer one-half teaspoon of powdered root in one cup of boiling water for thirty minutes. Cool. To improve flavor, add lemon or honey, if necessary. Take two tablespoons every few hours, up to one cup per day. As a tincture, take one teaspoon a day.

Precautions: This herb should be avoided during early pregnancy, so do not use it if there is any chance that you are pregnant. Any woman who has been advised by her doctor not to use oral contraceptives should also avoid this herb.

Chaste-tree *(Vitex agnus-castus)*

This herb is often recommended when a woman's body fails to produce a sufficient supply of progesterone; it helps to stimulate and normalize hormone levels. (Progesterone imbalances can be diagnosed using a blood test, or it may be indicated by a luteal phase dysfunction in the temperature chart; see pages 17-20 for information on temperature charting.) This herb is also used to prevent miscarriage and during recovery after hysterectomy.

Usage: Take ten drops of tincture in a cup of water each morning in the second half of the menstrual cycle. Look for a commercial preparation and follow package directions.

PRECAUTIONS: This herb can cause the sensation of insects crawling on the skin (formication).

Chi Shao Yao *(Paeonia lactiflora)*

This herb is used in traditional Chinese medicine for the treatment of female reproductive problems, including dysmenorrhea (lack of menstrual periods) caused by low levels of estrogen.

USAGE: Commercially prepared tinctures are available; follow package directions.

PRECAUTIONS: Estrogen-promoting herbs, such as chi shao yao, should be avoided by women with a personal or family history of breast or reproduction system cancers.

Dong Quai or Dom Kwai *(Angelica sinensis* or *Angelica polymorpha)*

This Chinese herb contains plant substances similar to female hormones; it strengthens the female reproductive organs and helps regulate menstrual periods, in addition to boosting fertility. It is the female counterpart to ginseng.

USAGE: For a tea, boil six cups of water and add one medium to large whole root. (For additional flavor, as well as for the overall health-enhancing benefits, you may also want to add one tablespoon of licorice root, one tablespoon of freshly grated ginger root, and a one-half-inch piece of cinnamon stick.) Simmer for twenty minutes. Drink two to three cups per day. Commercial preparations are also available; follow package directions.

PRECAUTIONS: It can cause breast tenderness.

Gotu Kola *(Centella asiatica* or *Hydrocotyle asiatica)*

This herb helps to achieve hormone balance and promote fertility. It also helps relax the nerves, enhance the immune system, speed wound healing, and improve blood circulation to the legs (which helps prevent varicose veins).

USAGE: For an infusion, use one-half teaspoon of herb per cup of boiling water. Simmer for twenty minutes, strain, and drink up to two cups a day. (You may want to add sugar, honey, or lemon to disguise the bitter taste.) Commercial preparations are also available; follow package directions. This herb is most effective when taken for four to six weeks, followed by a two-week break.

PRECAUTIONS: High doses can cause headaches, skin rash, or itching.

Nettle or Stinging Nettle *(Urtica dioica)*

Because of its high mineral and chlorophyll content, this herb is considered a powerful tonic for the hormone system. It also increases milk flow in nursing mothers. Native American women believed that drinking nettle tea during pregnancy would strengthen the fetus; they also used it to stop uterine bleeding after childbirth. Nettle is also used to treat hay fever symptoms, high blood pressure, and gout.

USAGE: For an infusion, add one to two teaspoons of dried herb to one cup of boiling water. Steep for fifteen minutes, strain, and drink up to two cups per day. As a tincture, use up to one teaspoon twice a day. Commercial preparations are also available; follow package directions.

PRECAUTIONS: Nettle can cause stomach upset, burning skin, and suppression of urine. Pregnant women should avoid this herb since it can cause uterine contractions; do not use it if there is any chance that you are pregnant.

Red Clover *(Trifolium pratense)*

In the body, red clover mimics the female hormone estrogen. It helps balance hormonal functions, and it is an excellent source of calcium and magnesium, which relax the nervous system and enhance fertility, in addition to offering a rich supply of many trace minerals essential for reproduction. In addition, red clover can help the body maintain a vaginal pH (acid/alkaline level) that favors conception. It is sometimes used to relieve menopausal symptoms, such as hot flashes, insomnia, and mood swings.

USAGE: Fresh red clover flowers can be added to salads, or a tablespoon of dried flowers can be added to rice during cooking. To prepare an infusion, add one to three teaspoons of dried flower to a cup of boiling water. Steep for fifteen minutes, strain, and drink up to three cups a day. (You may want to add one teaspoon of peppermint to improve the flavor.) Commercial preparations are also available; follow package directions.

PRECAUTIONS: Can cause stomach upset or diarrhea. Women with a history of breast or gynecological cancer should avoid red clover, as well as other herbs containing plant estrogens. Women with a history of heart disease or stroke should avoid this herb because it can increase the risk of developing blood clots.

Red Raspberry *(Rubus idaeus* or *Rubus strigosus)*

The leaves of this herb are rich in calcium and can relax and strengthen the uterus. Red raspberry is also used to treat diarrhea, nausea, and vomiting.

Usage: For an infusion, use one to two teaspoons of dried herb per cup of boiling water. Steep fifteen minutes, strain, and drink up to three cups a day. The infusion is especially beneficial when combined with red clover (use one teaspoon of red clover and one teaspoon of raspberry in two cups of water). Commercial preparations are also available; follow package directions.

Precautions: This is generally a safe herb. Avoid using it if you are pregnant, since it can stimulate the uterus during early pregnancy.

Skullcap *(Scutellaria lateriflora)*

This herb is widely used as a sedative and treatment for insomnia and nervousness, as well as a treatment for infertility. It is high in minerals that support a healthy nervous system. It is sometimes used in the treatment of premenstrual syndrome.

Usage: For an infusion, use one to two teaspoons of dried herb per cup of boiling water. Steep fifteen minutes, strain, and drink up to three cups a day. (You may want to add sugar, honey, or lemon to disguise the bitter flavor.) Commercial preparations are also available; follow package directions.

Precautions: Skullcap can cause confusion, muscle twitching, nausea, or diarrhea.

HIS

Ashwagandha *(Withania somnifera)*

This East Indian herb is considered a sexual tonic; it is good for promoting fertility and overcoming impotence. It is often referred to as Indian ginseng.

Usage: Add one teaspoon of root powder to boiled warm milk; take up to two cups a day. Commercial preparations are also available; follow package directions.

Precautions: Ashwagandha is generally regarded as a safe herb.

Burdock Root *(Arctium lappa)*

This herb is known to promote overall good health, in addition to boosting fertility by strengthening the male reproductive organs.

Usage: For a decoction, boil one teaspoon of root in three cups of water for thirty minutes. Drink up to three cups a day. In a tincture, take one-half to one teaspoon up to three times a day. Commercial preparations are also available; follow package directions. Combination products often include damiana and sarsaparilla (see page 83).

PRECAUTIONS: Burdock root can cause stomach upset.

Damiana *(Turnera diffusa aphrodisiaca)*

This herb helps stimulate testosterone production, increasing fertility and helping with impotence. Some experts believe that the herb slightly irritates the urethra, making the penis somewhat more sensitive. It is often used in combination with other herbs.

USAGE: For an infusion, use one teaspoon of powdered herb in one cup of water. Steep fifteen minutes; drink up to one cup per day. For a tincture, take up to one-half teaspoon three times a day. Commercial preparations are also available; follow package directions.

PRECAUTIONS: This herb should not be used by men with prostate problems, without a doctor's supervision.

Garlic *(Allium sativum)*

This herb is recommended for the treatment of impotence; it also helps balance both high and low blood pressure, lower blood cholesterol levels, lower blood sugar levels, and clear respiratory and digestive infections.

USAGE: Use garlic liberally in cooking. For an infusion, chop six cloves of garlic per cup of cool water and steep for six hours. For a tincture, soak one cup of crushed garlic cloves in one quart of brandy; shake daily for two weeks, then take up to three tablespoons a day. Commercial preparations are also available; follow package directions.

PRECAUTIONS: Garlic has anti-clotting properties; it should be avoided by people with clotting disorders without a doctor's supervision. It can also cause stomach upset.

Ginkgo *(Ginkgo biloba)*

This herb helps relieve impotence and erectile dysfunction caused by damage to the arteries in the penis because it is a peripheral vasodilator. (It increases blood flow to the penis—as well as other veins—without changing systemic blood pressure.) According to a study published in the *Journal of Urology*, half of the men taking 60 milligrams of ginkgo daily regained erections within a year.

USAGE: This herb is typically available only in commercial preparations; follow package directions.

PRECAUTIONS: Ginkgo can cause irritability and restlessness. Since it can inhibit blood clotting, it should be avoided by people with clotting disorders.

Ginseng *(Panax quinquefoliaus*/American ginseng; *Panax ginseng*/Chinese ginseng; *Eleutherococcus senticosus*/Siberian ginseng)

This herb boosts sperm counts by helping men manage their stress and anxiety; it also helps promote overall health and normalize blood pressure. Ginseng has a long history as a male "tonic," and American Indians used to mix ginseng into love potions. Animal studies have found that this herb can promote growth of the testes, increase sperm formation, raise testosterone levels, and increase the frequency of sexual activity.

USAGE: To make a decoction, add one-half teaspoon of dried root powder to one cup of boiling water. Simmer ten minutes; drink up to two cups a day. Commercial products are widely available; look for products made of whole, unprocessed roots that are at least six years old (the medicinal properties are found only in mature roots). Follow package directions.

Precautions: Ginseng can cause insomnia or breast tenderness. Since it has anti-clotting properties, ginseng should be avoided by people with clotting disorders.

Hawthorn *(Crataegus oxyacantha)*

This herb helps to strengthen the cardiovascular and circulatory systems, improving blood flow to the penis and throughout the body. The Greeks and Romans associated this herb with marriage and fertility.

Usage: For an infusion, add two teaspoons of crushed dried leaves to one cup of boiling water. Steep twenty minutes. Strain and drink up to two cups a day. (You may want to add lemon, sugar, or honey to mask the bitter flavor.) Commercial preparations are also available; follow package directions.

Precautions: Can cause low blood pressure and fainting; people with heart problems should consult a physician before using hawthorn.

Licorice *(Glycyrrhiza glabra)*

This herb boosts sperm counts by helping men manage their stress and anxiety; it also helps promote overall health, normalize blood pressure, and heal ulcers and other gastrointestinal-tract problems.

USAGE: To make a decoction, add one-half teaspoon of powdered herb to one cup of boiling water. Simmer ten minutes; drink up to two cups a day. Licorice—also known as "sweet root"—is fifty times sweeter than sugar, so you shouldn't need to enhance the flavor. As a tincture, use one-half to one teaspoon up to two times a day. Commercial products are also available; follow package directions.

PRECAUTIONS: Licorice can cause stomach upset or diarrhea. It is not recommended for people with high blood pressure.

Pygeum *(Pygeum africanum)*

This herb may be helpful when diminished prostate secretion plays a role in male-factor infertility. Pygeum has been shown to increase the volume of prostatic secretions and to improve the composition of the seminal fluid.

USAGE: For an infusion, add one teaspoon of herb to one cup of boiling water. Steep for twenty minutes. Strain and drink one cup per day. Commercial products are also available; follow package directions.

Precautions: Pygeum is generally considered a safe herb.

Saw Palmetto *(Serenoa repens)*

This herb strengthens the male reproductive system and enhances the male sex hormones. It also improves overall health.

Usage: For an infusion, add one teaspoon of herb to one cup of boiling water. Steep for twenty minutes. Strain and drink one cup per day. Commercial products are also available; follow package directions.

Precautions: Saw palmetto is generally considered a safe herb.

Yohimbe *(Pausinystalia yohimba)*

The bark of the evergreen African yohimbe tree has earned a reputation as an herbal aphrodisiac, and it can be very effective in the treatment of impotence and erectile dysfunction. In fact, yohimbe is the source of yohimbine, a prescription drug used to treat impotence. Yohimbe should not be used on a regular and ongoing basis because it can elevate blood pressure; do not use this herb for more than two weeks at a time. This herb has been found to be ineffective when impotence stems from organic nerve trouble.

USAGE: For a decoction, simmer one ounce of bark in two cups of water for five to ten minutes. Strain and drink one to two cups 15 to 30 minutes before making love. (You may want to add 1 gram of vitamin C per cup of decoction to reduce the likelihood of stomach upset.) Commercial preparations are also available; follow package directions.

PRECAUTIONS: Yohimbe can cause dangerous low blood pressure; this herb should not be used by people with hypotension. It can also cause nausea.

COUPLES

False Unicorn Root *(Chamaelirium luteum)*

This herb has earned a reputation of being very effective in the treatment of infertility by correcting hormone imbalances. It is a uterine stimulant that can be useful in the treatment of irregular periods in women; it is also useful in treating impotence in men. It is believed to have a beneficial effect on the ovaries, kidneys, and bladder, and it is sometimes used to prevent miscarriage. Commercial products often combine false unicorn root with black cohosh (see page 68) and wild yam (see page 84).

USAGE: It is available in commercial combination tinctures and capsules; follow package directions. (Herbalists have been known to warn couples taking this herb for other medical conditions of its potency in promoting fertility.)

PRECAUTIONS: False unicorn root can cause nausea and vomiting.

Sarsaparilla *(Smilax officinalis* and *Smilax febrifuga)*

This herb boosts fertility by stimulating the production of progesterone in women and testosterone in men. It also has diuretic properties. Caribbean and North American Indians used the herb to keep people young, vigorous, and potent.

USAGE: For a decoction, use one to two teaspoons of powdered root per cup of water. Bring to a boil and simmer for fifteen minutes. Drink up to three cups a day. In a tincture, take one-fourth to one-half teaspoon up to three times a day. Commercial preparations are also available; follow package directions.

PRECAUTIONS: Sarsaparilla can cause stomach upset and a burning sensation in the mouth. Because of its diuretic properties, women should avoid sarsaparilla if there is any chance that they could be pregnant.

Wild Yam *(Dioscorea villosa)*

This herb contains hormonelike substances that are very similar to progesterone. In fact, it was used to make the original contraceptive pills before synthetic hormones were available. In women, wild yam can help normalize hormone levels. In men, it helps relax peripheral blood vessels, which can improve blood flow to the penis.

USAGE: For an infusion, add one teaspoon of dried herb to one cup of boiling water. Steep twenty minutes; strain and drink up to one cup per day. Commercial preparations are also available; follow package directions.

PRECAUTIONS: Since it stimulates hormone production, this herb should be avoided by people with a history of reproductive disorders. It should also be discontinued once pregnancy has been achieved.

Try One or More Herbs for Stress

Each of the following herbs listed can help reduce anxiety and stress, which can contribute to infertility.

(For more information on stress and infertility, see Chapter 7, "Mind-Body Connection," on page 123.)

USAGE: For an infusion, use one to two teaspoons for dried herb per cup of boiling water. Steep for fifteen minutes. Strain and drink up to three cups a day. Add honey or sugar to mask the bitter flavor, if necessary.

✷ **Kava Kava** *(Kava Kava)*

This herb is a nervine relaxant, which can be used to soothe frazzled nerves.

PRECAUTIONS: This herb can cause headaches or nausea.

✷ **St. John's wort** *(Hypericum perforatum)*

This herb has been used for more than two thousand years in the treatment of insomnia, anxiety, and depression; it is also used to boost the immune system and to help with wound healing.

PRECAUTIONS: Do not use when taking amphetamines, narcotics, diet pills, asthma inhalants, nasal decongestants, or cold or hay fever remedies. Also avoid beer, wine, coffee, salami, yogurt, chocolate, and smoked or pickled foods. Avoid sun to prevent sunburn.

❋ **Skullcap** *(Scutellaria lateriflora)*

The Chinese have used this herb as a tranquilizer for centuries. Modern herbalists use it for insomnia, nervous tension, and premenstrual syndrome. It is used in many commercial sleep preparations in Europe.

PRECAUTIONS: Skullcap can cause confusion, muscle twitching, nausea, or diarrhea.

❋ **Valerian** *(Valeriana officinalis)*

This herb is the active ingredient in more than one hundred over-the-counter tranquilizers and insomnia remedies in Europe. It has been used for centuries both as a "nervine tonic" and anticonvulsant.

PRECAUTIONS: Valerian can cause headaches, giddiness, blurred vision, nausea, or restlessness.

❋ **Vervain** *(Perbena officinalis)*

This herb is used as a tranquilizer, pain reliever, fever reducer, and expectorant. It acts like a mild aspirin, relieving stress and pain and reducing inflammation.

PRECAUTIONS: This herb can lower heart rate; it should be avoided by anyone with congestive heart failure or a history of heart disease. It also should be avoided by asthmatics and people with respiratory problems.

FERTILITY CHECKLIST

HERS

- ❑ Black cohosh
- ❑ Chaste tree
- ❑ Chi shao yao
- ❑ Dong quai
- ❑ Gotu kola
- ❑ Nettle
- ❑ Red clover
- ❑ Red raspberry
- ❑ Skullcap

HIS

- ❑ Ashwagandha
- ❑ Burdock root
- ❑ Damiana
- ❑ Garlic
- ❑ Ginkgo
- ❑ Ginseng
- ❑ Hawthorn
- ❑ Licorice
- ❑ Pygeum
- ❑ Saw palmetto
- ❑ Yohimbe

COUPLES

- ❑ False unicorn root
- ❑ Sarsaparilla
- ❑ Wild yam
- ❑ Herbs for stress:
    - Kava Kava
    - St. John's wort
    - Skullcap
    - Valerian
    - Vervain

5
Homeopathy: Baby Doses for Big Results

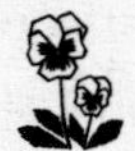

Homeopathy, like conception itself, remains something of a mystery. Researchers have documented and even witnessed the process of egg fertilization and human conception, but the essence of the creation of life remains incomprehensible. In much the same way, homeopaths have learned how to use homeopathy in the treatment of medical problems and seen evidence of its healing potential, but the essence of its medical power remains unknown.

The practice of homeopathy was developed in the late eighteenth century by Dr. Samuel Hahnemann (1755–1843), a German physician who had been trained in the practice of conventional medicine. At the time, mainstream medicine included a number of crude and sometimes harmful medical practices, such as bloodletting, induced vomiting, and the use of massive doses of poorly understood drugs. Hahnemann, on the other hand, believed in the healing powers of nutrition and exercise (this was a radical idea at the time). He experimented with other methods of treatment, often testing potential remedies on himself. In one experiment, Hahnemann tested cinchona (also known as Peruvian bark), which is the natural source of quinine. When he took small doses of cinchona, Hahnemann developed the symptoms of malaria: fever, chills, thirst, and a throbbing headache. He hypothesized that cinchona would be effective in treating malaria because of its ability to produce similar symptoms to those of the disease.

The results of this experiment led to Hahnemann's first theory, the Law of Similars, or "like cures like." According to the theory, certain illnesses can be cured by giving the sick person minuscule doses of natural substances—plants, minerals, chemicals, and animal substances—that would produce the symptoms of the disease in a healthy person.

As one might expect, Hahnemann found that higher concentrations of substances caused more side effects. However, in further experiments he found that he could dilute a medication and still preserve its healing powers through a pharmacological process he called "potentization." Hahnemann determined that by repeatedly diluting a substance with distilled water or alcohol and shaking it vigorously between each dilution, he could increase the potency of the medicine. These findings resulted in Hahnemann's theory, the Law of Infinitesimals, which states that the smaller the dose of active ingredient, the more potent the cure.

Homeopathy was put to the test in dealing with epidemic diseases, such as cholera, typhoid, yellow fever, and scarlet fever. The success of the treatment led to widespread interest in its practice. The first homeopathy college opened in Philadelphia in 1836, and eight years later a group of homeopaths formed the American Institute of Homeopathy, the first national medical organization in the country. By the end of the nineteenth century, there were fifteen thousand homeopaths and twenty-two schools of homeopathy nationwide. Homeopathy also flourished and continues to thrive in Europe, particularly in Great Britain, where the Queen of England has her own homeopathic physician and the British National Health Service covers homeopathic procedures.

In the United States, however, homeopathy rapidly fell out of favor. At the end of the nineteenth century one out of every five American doctors practiced homeopathy, but by the middle of the twentieth century the American practice of homeopathy had all but disappeared. The discovery of antibiotics and other advances in modern medicine lured people to support a more "scientific" approach to healing. Professional medical groups, influenced by these developments, began to expel physicians who practiced homeopathy or consulted with homeopaths. Hahnemann's theories have never been accepted by scientifically oriented physicians in the United States, who charge that homeopathic remedies are placebos.

Only recently has the homeopathic revival begun in the United States, in part because skeptics have been quieted by a number of studies showing that homeopathic remedies do help in the healing process. In 1991 the *British Medical Journal* tried to put the question to rest by publishing an analysis of 105 clinical studies involving the efficacy of homeopathy. More than eighty of the studies showed that the homeopathic treatment was more effective than a placebo.

No one knows exactly why homeopathy works, but some experts theorize that the repeated dilution and shaking establishes a certain electrochemical pattern in the water. Then, when someone takes a homeopathic remedy, the electrochemical pattern in the remedy affects the electrochemical pattern of the water in the human body. Other experts suggest that the potentization changes the electromagnetic fields in the body in some subtle way. Both of these theories involve energy changes at a subatomic level, a level that we can never see and few of us will ever understand.

Additional research will undoubtedly be conducted to prove or disprove various theories about homeopathy. In the meantime, homeopaths and open-minded patients will continue to use the treatments, not because they understand how they work but because they know from firsthand experience that they do.

TREAT THE PERSON, NOT THE DISEASE

Homeopaths and traditional doctors approach healing from different points of view. Homeopaths believe illness is not localized in one organ or manifested in one symptom, so when prescribing treatment they consider the entire person, both mind and body. While traditional physicians attempt to manage illness by relieving symptoms, homeopaths consider physical symptoms positive signs that the body is hard at work defending and healing itself. Rather than trying to eliminate symptoms, homeopathic remedies sometimes even aggravate symptoms for a short period of time as they stimulate the body's self-healing mechanism.

PRACTICING HOMEOPATHY

Unlike other medical practices, the selection of the appropriate homeopathic remedy varies from patient to patient, depending on the patient profile and the specific symptoms that are present. When you use the right remedy, it will work quickly and you can discontinue treatment. The wrong remedy will cause no harm, but it will not help you conceive.

Homeopathic remedies are prepared according to standards of the United States Homeopathy Pharmacopoeia and come in a variety of potencies, based on the strength of dilution. The three most common forms of remedies are the mother tincture, x potencies, and c potencies:

Mother Tincture

The mother tincture is an alcohol-based extract of a specific substance; tinctures are usually used topically rather than internally.

X Potencies

The x represent the Roman numeral 10. In homeopathic remedies with x potencies, the mother tincture has been diluted to one part in ten (one drop of tincture to every nine drops of alcohol). The number before the x tells how many times the mother tincture has been diluted. For example, a 12x potency represents 12 dilutions of one in ten. According to homeopathic theory, the more the substance is diluted, the more potent it becomes, so a remedy with a 30x potency is considered stronger or more potent than one with a 12x potency.

C Potencies

The c represents the Roman number 100. Homeopathic remedies with a c potency have been diluted to one part in 100 (one drop of tincture to every ninety-nine drops of alcohol), making them much stronger than x potencies. Again, the number before the c represents the number of dilutions. A 3c potency represents a substance that has been diluted to one part in one hundred three times; by the time 3c is reached, the dilution is one part per million.

Homeopathic remedies come in a number of forms, but the most common are lactose (milk sugar) pilules and liquids. When you are taking homeopathic pilules, one or two of the tiny, poppyseed-sized globules are placed on the tongue to dissolve. When you are taking a liquid homeopathic remedy, a single drop of the substance is placed under the tongue.

Tips for Usage

- When taking homeopathic remedies, avoid coffee, alcohol, tobacco, minty flavorings, highly perfumed cosmetics and toiletries, and strong-smelling household cleaners. These strong odors and flavors can overpower the subtle effects of the treatment.
- Take homeopathic remedies between meals, at least a half-hour after eating. They should not be taken when your mouth tastes of toothpaste, tobacco, spicy foods, or other flavors.
- Store homeopathic remedies in a cool, dark, dry place free of strong-smelling substances.

Q&A

Is it okay to use homeopathic remedies in conjunction with herbal remedies?

Yes. However, you should wait at least a half-hour after taking an herbal remedy before using a homeopathic treatment.

Is it harmful to use the wrong homeopathic remedy?

Using the wrong remedy will cause no harm, but it will do nothing to enhance your fertility. Because the amount of active ingredient in a homeopathic remedy is so small, side effects from these treatments are virtually nonexistent.

When should I take a homeopathic remedy?

Most of the homeopathic remedies discussed in this chapter can be taken for one week (those used for uterine problems can be taken for three weeks). A woman should take the remedy during the start of her menstrual cycle (with the first day of bleeding). A man should take a remedy several days prior to the target date of conception. If you use a commercially prepared product with different directions, follow the information provided on the label.

Where can I find homeopathic remedies?

Homeopathic remedies are available at many health food stores, as well as specialized pharmacies (see pages 186-189 for a listing of manufacturers).

Is there any evidence that homeopathy really works?

Researchers have not studied the efficacy of homeopathy in the treatment of infertility. However, a number of studies published in respected medical journals have shown that homeopathic remedies work in the treatment of other medical problems. Consider some of the evidence:

- A British medical journal published an analysis of 105 clinical studies involving the efficacy of homeopathy. The homeopathic treatment was found to be more effective than a placebo in eighty-one of the studies. Critics of homeopathy charged that many of the studies were poorly designed, but a review of twenty-six of the better-controlled studies found that fifteen demonstrated the benefit of homeopathic treatments.
- 1994: A study published in the British medical journal *The Lancet* found that homeopathic treatment outperformed a placebo in bringing relief to twenty-eight patients who were allergic to dust mites.
- 1994: The peer-reviewed American medical journal *Pediatrics* reported that among eighty-one children in Nicaragua treated for diarrhea, those given a homeopathic treatment in addition to the standard oral rehydration therapy got well faster than those who got the standard treatment alone. Among the children in the control group, the diarrhea lasted an average of four days, but in the group receiving the homeopathic treatment it lasted two and a half days.

HERS

✸ **Causticum 30c:** Use this remedy if you experience a loss of interest in sex following your period, or if your vagina feels sore and irritated. Take one dose every twelve hours for up to one week.

Full Latin name: *Causticum hahnemnni.*

Source: calcium oxide and potassium bisulfate.

✸ **Conium 30c:** Use this remedy if your breasts feel tender and swollen, or if you experience a loss of interest in sex. Take one dose every twelve hours for up to one week.

Full Latin name: *Conium maculatum.*

Source: hemlock (fresh plant when in flower).

✸ **Ignatia 30c:** Use this remedy if you are experiencing grief or loss related to a previous relationship. Take one dose every twelve hours for up to one week.

Full Latin name: *Ignatia amara* or *Strychnos ignatia.*

Source: St. Ignatius' bean (seed pods).

✸ **Lycopodium 30c:** Use this remedy if you experience vaginal dryness and tenderness on the right side of your lower abdomen. Take one dose every twelve hours for up to one week.

Full Latin name: *Lycopodium clavatum.*

Source: wolf's claw club moss (spores).

✸ **Phosphoric acidum 30c:** Use this remedy if you

feel apathetic or indifferent about having sex with your partner. Take one dose every twelve hours for up to one week.

Full Latin name: *Phosphoricum acidum.*

Source: phosphoric acid.

✹ **Pulsatilla 30c:** Use this remedy if you feel anxious about having intercourse, especially if you tend to be emotional and weepy. Take one dose every twelve hours for up to five days.

Full Latin name: *Pulsatilla nigricans.*

Source: wind flower, pasque flower (whole fresh plant when in flower).

✹ **Sabina 30c:** Use this remedy if you have been pregnant and experienced a miscarriage during the first trimester. Take one dose every twelve hours for up to one week.

Full Latin name: *Juniperus sabina.*

Source: savin juniper (new leaves at tips of branches).

✹ **Sepia 30c:** Use this remedy if you have irregular periods, or if you have an aversion to sex. Take one dose every twelve hours for up to one week.

Full Latin name: *Sepia officinalis.*

Source: cuttlefish ink.

If uterus problems accompany infertility:

✹ **Aurum muriaticum 6c:** Use this remedy if your uterus feels swollen and painful, or if you feel spasms or contractions in your vagina. Take one dose four times daily for up to three weeks.

Full Latin name: *Aurum muriaticum.*

Source: gold chloride.

✹ **Calcarea iodata 6c:** Use this remedy if you have had small fibroids accompanied by yellowish vaginal discharge. Take one dose four times daily for up to three weeks.

Full Latin name: *Calcarea iodata.*

Source: calcium iodide.

✹ **Fraxinus 6c:** Use this remedy if you have painful cramps during your periods and thin, brown discharge from your vagina between periods. Take one dose four times daily for up to three weeks.

Full Latin name: *Fraxinus americanus.*

Source: white ash (bark).

✹ **Kali iodatum 6c:** Use this remedy if you experience uterine cramping or squeezing during periods. Take one dose four times daily for up to three weeks.

Full Latin name: *Kali iodatum.*

Source: potassium iodide.

✹ **Silicea 6c:** Use this remedy if you tend to have

heavy menstrual flow and spotting between periods. Take one dose four times daily for up to three weeks.

Full Latin name: *Silicea terra*.

Source: flint.

HIS

✹ **Agnus 30c:** Use this remedy if you cannot achieve and maintain an erection, or if you experience an overall lack of energy. Take one dose every twelve hours for up to one week.

Full Latin name: *Agnus castus*.

Source: chaste-tree (ripe berries).

✹ **Conium 30c:** Use this remedy if you cannot achieve and maintain an erection and you experience cramping and coldness in your legs. Take one dose every twelve hours for up to one week.

Full Latin name: *Conium maculatum*.

Source: hemlock (fresh plant when in flower).

✹ **Graphites 30c:** Use this remedy if you have lost interest in sex, if you experience premature ejaculation, or if you cannot achieve ejaculation. Take one dose every twelve hours for up to five days.

Full Latin name: *Graphites*.

Source: black lead from finest drawing pencils.

✹ **Lycopodium 30c:** Use this remedy if you have a

strong desire for sex, but the experience is thwarted by insecurity and anxiety about failure. Take one dose every twelve hours for up to one week.

Full Latin name: *Lycopodium clavatum.*

Source: wolf's claw club moss (spores).

✷ **Nitric acidum 30c:** Use this remedy if you have little or no interest in sex; you may also feel irritable, self-castigating, and very sensitive to criticism. Take one dose every twelve hours for up to five days.

Full Latin name: *Nitricum acidum.*

Source: Nitric acid.

✷ **Nux 30c:** Use this remedy if you experience ejaculation problems; you may also feel short-tempered and impatient. Take one dose every twelve hours for up to one week.

Full Latin name: *Strychnos nux vomica.*

Source: poison nut tree (seeds).

✷ **Phosphoric acidum 30c:** Use this remedy if you have little or no interest in sex. Take one dose every twelve hours for up to five days.

Full Latin name: *Phosphoricum acidum.*

Source: phosphoric acid.

✷ **Sepia 30c:** Use this remedy if you have no interest in sex and feel a "dragging" sensation in your genitals. Take one dose every twelve hours for up to one week.

Full Latin name: *Sepia officinalis.*

Source: cuttlefish ink.

FERTILITY CHECKLIST

HERS

Consider using *one* of the following homeopathic remedies:

❏ Causticum 30c
❏ Conium 30c
❏ Ignatia 30c
❏ Lycopodium 30c
❏ Phosphoric acidum 30c
❏ Pulsatilla 30c
❏ Sabina 30c
❏ Sepia 30c
❏ Aurum muriaticum 6c
❏ Calcarea iodata 6c
❏ Fraxinus 6c
❏ Kali iodata 6c
❏ Silicea 6c

HIS

Consider using *one* of the following homeopathic remedies:

❏ Agnus 30c
❏ Conium 30c
❏ Graphites 30c
❏ Lycopodium 30c
❏ Nitric acidium 30c
❏ Nux 30c
❏ Phosphoric acidium 30c
❏ Sepia 30c

6
Acupressure: Hands-on Healing

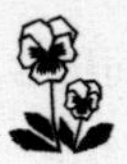

For more than five thousand years, healers have relied on the soothing touch of acupressure to balance the body's energy and correct ailments and illnesses, including sexual dysfunction, gynecological complaints, and infertility.

The ancient healing arts of acupressure and acupuncture involve the use of either fingertip pressure or fine needles to activate a network of key pressure points, promoting muscle relaxation and increasing blood circulation. Healers have refined the techniques over the centuries, as they have observed and recorded the relationships between healing and touch at various points on the body.

The points used for acupressure and acupuncture are the same. Studies have demonstrated that acupuncture has been successful in the treatment of infertility. According to *The Shanghai Journal of Acupuncture*, acupuncturists stimulated key fertility points for thirty to forty minutes every other day, beginning on the tenth day of the menstrual cycle. Fully 57 percent of the women in the study had conceived within two courses of treatment. Of course, acupuncture offers a more intense form of stimulation than acupressure, but you may be able to evoke a healing response on your own by practicing acupressure at home. If you would like to consult an acupuncturist, see pages 189-191 for information on finding a qualified professional.

UNDERSTANDING ACUPRESSURE

Acupressurists and acupuncturists use two types of pressure points: local points (pressure points located where the pain occurs) and trigger points (pressure points located far from the site where the pain occurs). Trigger points stimulate a response in distant parts of the body because they lie along a network of electrical channels (called meridians) that run throughout the body. Ancient Chinese healers have identified twelve major meridians, each named after or corresponding to a different organ, such as large intestine, small intestine, or bladder.

The meridians connect the acupressure points in what can be considered an invisible wiring system for the flow of bioelectrical impulses or the body's "essential life energy," known as *chi* or *qi* in Chinese. Traditional Chinese healers believe that chi comes in two opposite but complementary forms, yin (passive energy) and yang (active energy). When these two types of chi are balanced, the body is in harmony and in good health. When someone suffers from an injury or illness, however, chi falls out of balance. To correct an imbalance, you need to stimulate one or more of the appropriate pressure points.

Western healers may not accept the traditional explanation for how acupressure works, but the evidence shows that it does. Research shows that acupressure stimulates the release of endorphins, the body's natural painkillers and mood and immune-system regulators. In fact, studies have shown that endorphin levels in the brain double thirty minutes after a session of acupuncture. The evidence is compelling enough that the U.S. Food and Drug Administration approved its use in the treatment of several medical problems.

Skeptics have argued that the benefits attributed to acupressure and acupuncture should be attributed instead to the placebo effect, or the ability of a patient's expectations to influence his or her reported experience of healing. However, studies have shown that acupuncture proves effective in pain control 55 to 85 percent of the time, much more than can be explained by the placebo effect alone.

While not intended to replace conventional medical care, acupuncture (in the hands of a trained professional) or acupressure (as a method of self-care) may help to boost your fertility.

GETTING TO THE POINT

To the beginner, acupressure can seem complex and intimidating. But once you begin to experiment with the technique, it will become very natural, and you will be able to enjoy its relaxing and healing benefits.

To help you get to the point—or more precisely to each of the body's 365 named and numbered acupressure points—experts have developed elaborate maps of the human body, using joints, muscles, and indentations in the bones as physical landmarks. The body is symmetrical, and most acupressure points are bilateral, occurring on both sides of the body. Except when an acupressure point falls on the midline of the body, acupressure should be applied to points on both sides.

When practicing acupressure, you'll know you've found the correct point (also known as *tsubo*) if you feel a tingle, "charge," or electrical impulse when you apply direct pressure; the point may also feel tender. In most cases, these points are located along the bones or beneath the major muscle groups.

After locating the correct spot, you will use your thumbs, middle fingers, palms, or the sides of your hands to apply firm, steady pressure. Your finger should be held at a right angle to the body. Start with a gentle touch and gradually push harder, until you feel a deep, even pressure, but not pain. Remember that fleshy parts of the body can withstand firmer pressure than bony areas. During an acupressure session, work the points on both sides of the body to maintain balance and harmony in your body.

Three to five minutes of steady, firm pressure works best, but as little as one minute can begin to promote healing and quiet the nervous system. At the end of an acupressure session, you should feel relaxed and invigorated, but don't expect that the pain will subside and your symptoms will disappear immediately. Acupressure isn't a matter of pressing a button and exacting a "cure." For the best results, plan on spending fifteen minutes or so working through your acupressure points two or three times a day.

HINTS FOR HANDS-ON HEALING

- Before starting your acupressure session, take a few minutes to relax and get focused. If possible, settle into a quiet, warm, and well-ventilated room. Start with some deep breathing to help you relax.
- If you are practicing acupressure on yourself, some points will be difficult to press without straining. To reach points on your back, place a soft tennis ball on a carpet and smoothly roll over onto it while supporting most of your weight on your elbows. If this is impossible to do without discomfort, either skip the point or ask your partner for help.
- Keep your fingernails short to avoid scratching or poking your skin.
- Make sure to smoothly and gradually increase the pressure, and smoothly and gradually release the pressure. Avoid sharp pokes or jabs.
- Remember that acupressure should not hurt. If a point feels painful to the touch, gradually release the pressure and move to another point.
- Avoid contact with areas that have been burned, bruised, cut, sprained, or infected. If the surrounding area is not too tender, consider applying pressure to the points near the injury to stimulate blood flow and to promote healing in the area.

- If you feel particularly stiff or tense before a session, consider soaking in a hot bath or applying a hot water bottle or heating pad to the affected area before beginning treatment.
- If possible, wait at least an hour after eating before practicing acupressure. Also avoid scheduling your acupressure sessions during times when you feel particularly hungry.

HERS

To help boost your fertility, use one or more of the following acupressure points.

Conception Vessel 3

Apply pressure on the midline of the lower abdomen, about one hand width below the belly button and one thumb width above the top of the pubic bone. In addition to improving fertility, this point helps to strengthen the reproductive organs, regulate menstruation, and reduce vaginal discharge.

Governing Vessel 23

This point is located along the midline of the scalp in line with the top of the nose and about one finger width inside your hairline. In addition to improving fertility, this point helps to tone the uterus and balance the hormonal system.

Large Intestine 4

Apply pressure to the end of the crease made when the index finger and thumb are pressed together. In addition to improving fertility, this point helps to ease abdominal pain and cramping and relieve constipation and other gastrointestinal complaints.

Spleen 6

This point is located on the inside of the leg, four finger widths above the tip of the ankle bone and just inside the tibia (the leg bone). In addition to improving fertility, this point helps to regulate menstruation and ease genital pain.

Spleen 8

Apply pressure on the inside of the lower leg four finger widths below the knee in the depression underneath the bone. In addition to improving fertility, this point helps to remove blockage in the lower abdomen and regulate menstruation.

ACUPRESSURE POINTS ON THE FACE

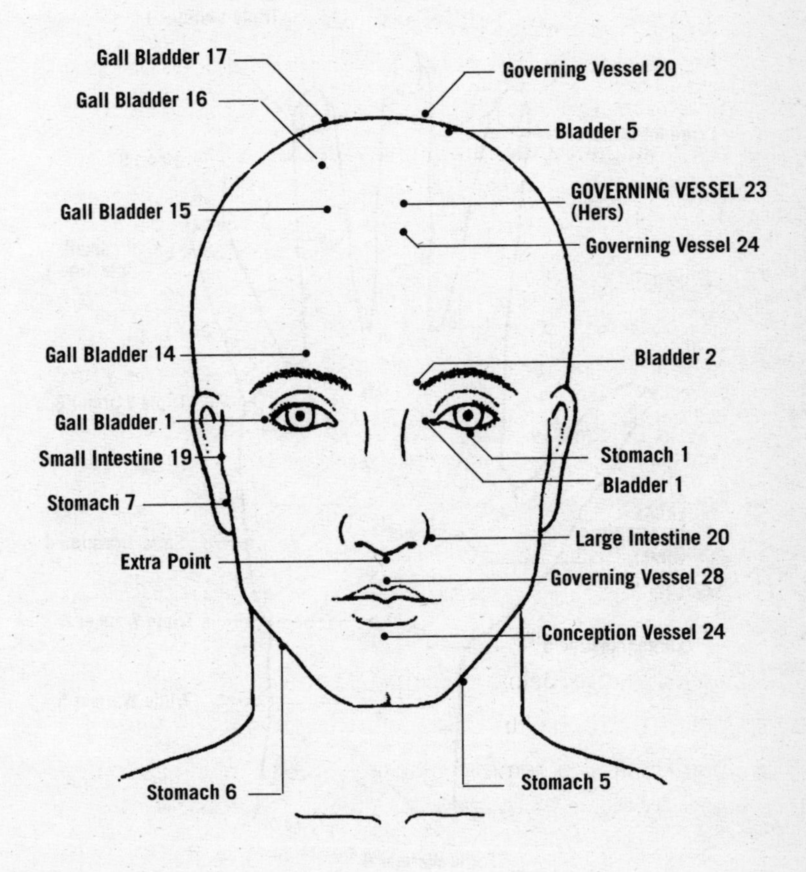

ACUPRESSURE POINTS ON THE HAND

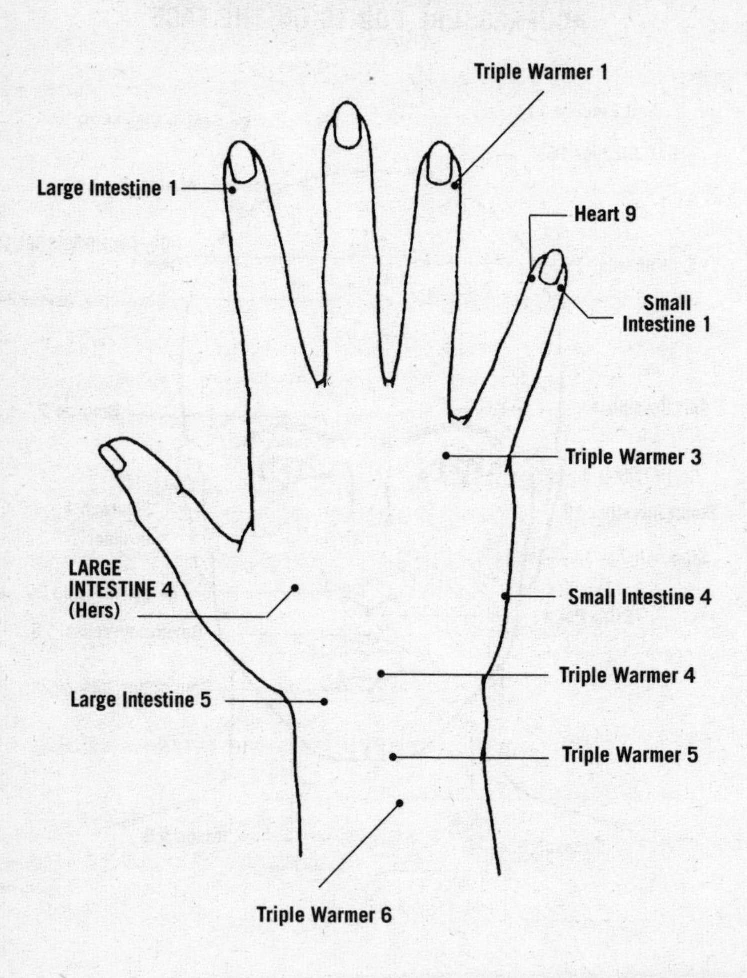

Spleen 10

This point is located on the inside edge of the top of the knee, where you can feel the muscle move when the knee is flexed. In addition to improving fertility, this point helps to improve blood circulation and relieve menstrual pain.

HIS

To help boost your fertility, use one or more of the following acupressure points.

Kidney 1

Apply pressure on the center of the sole of the foot, at the base of the ball of the foot, between the two pads. This point helps to relieve impotency.

COUPLES

To help boost your fertility, use one or more of the following acupressure points.

Bladder 23

This point is located on the lower back at waist level (in line with the belly button), two finger widths away from the spine. In addition to promoting fertility, this

ACUPRESSURE POINTS ON THE BOTTOM OF THE FOOT

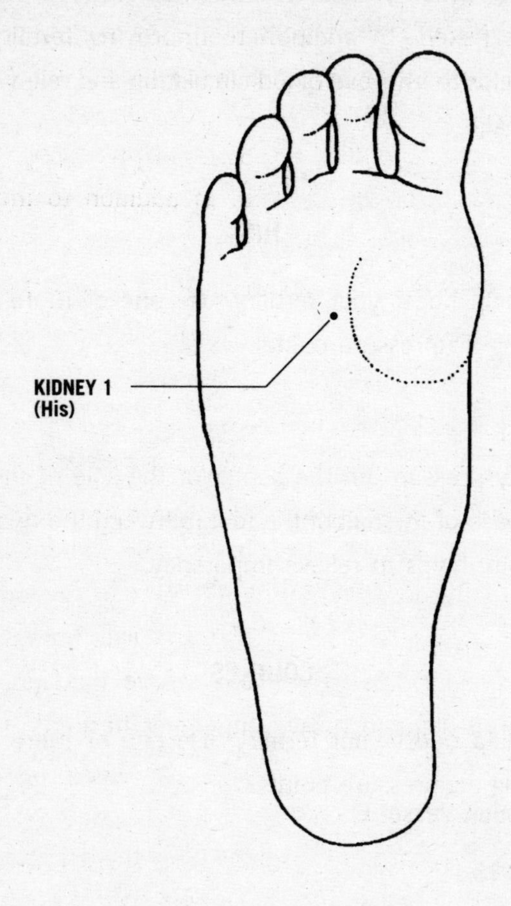

point helps to relieve lower-back pain and ease fatigue. It also helps with impotency and problems with ejaculation in men, and helps to regulate menstrual periods and reduce vaginal discharge in women.

Bladder 32

Apply pressure at the base of the spine, level with the second holes of the sacrum. In addition to improving fertility, this point helps to improve blood flow in the uterus, relieve lower-back pain, and regulate periods in women. It also helps overcome impotence in men.

Conception Vessel 4

This point is located on the midline of the abdomen, four finger widths below the belly button. In addition to improving fertility, this point helps to strengthen the abdominal muscles and tone the reproductive organs in men and women. It also helps to regulate menstruation, reduce vaginal discharge, and relieve incontinence in women. It helps to relieve impotence in men.

Conception Vessel 6

Apply pressure on the midline of the abdomen, two finger widths below the belly button (just above conception vessel 4). In addition to improving fertility, this point helps to strengthen the abdominal muscles and tone the

ACUPRESSURE POINTS ON THE BACK OF THE BODY

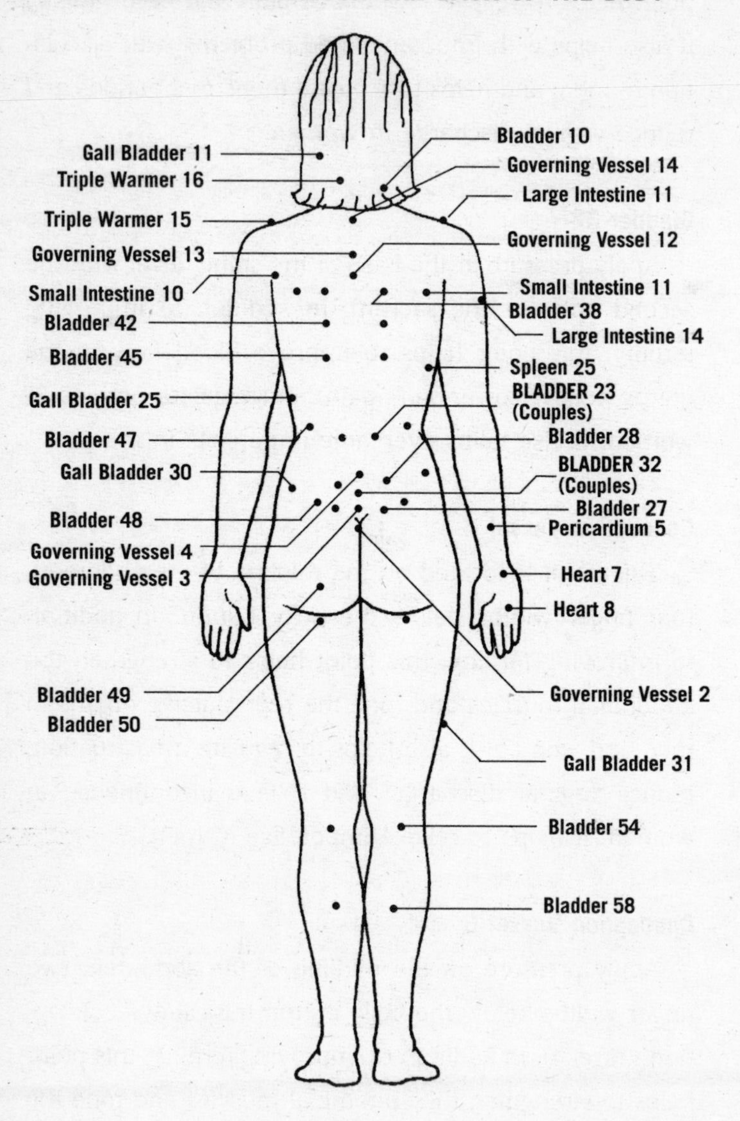

ACUPRESSURE POINTS ON THE FRONT OF THE BODY

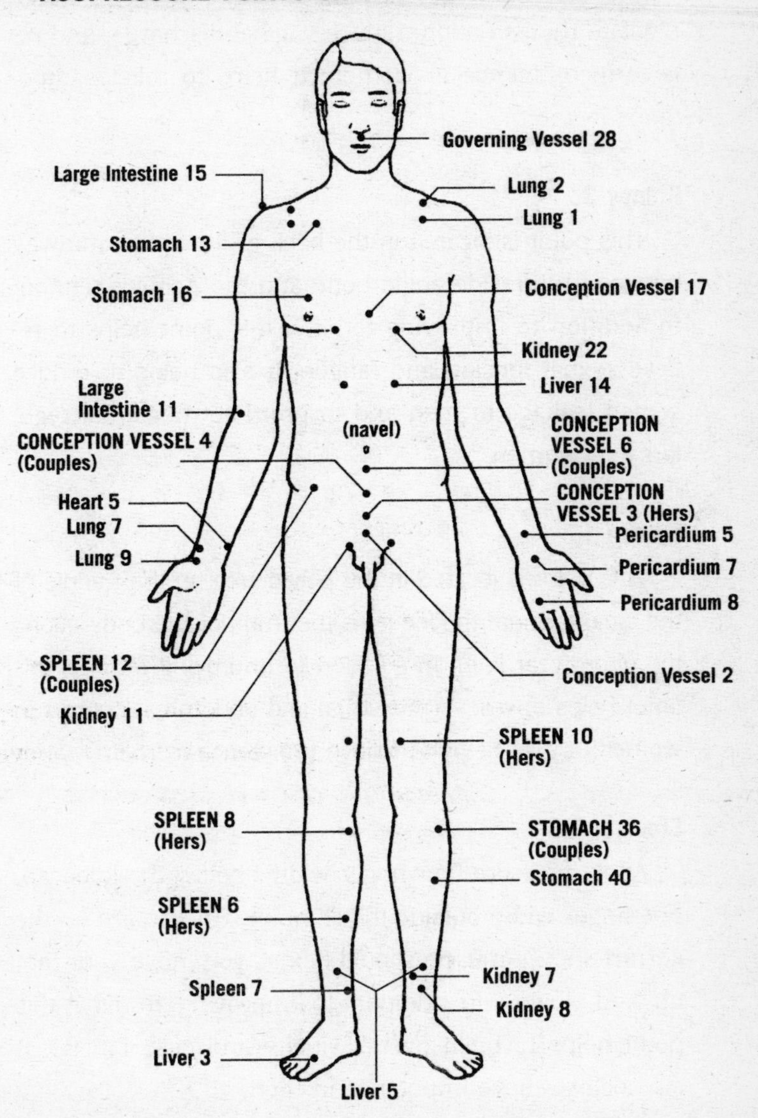

reproductive organs in men and women. It also helps regulate menstruation, reduce vaginal discharge, and relieve incontinence in women. It helps to relieve impotence in men.

Kidney 3

This point is located in the back of the ankle, midway between the inside ankle bone and the Achilles tendon. In addition to improving fertility, this point helps to relieve sexual tension and fatigue. It also helps to reduce semen leakage in men and to promote menstrual regularity in women.

Spleen 12

This point is located in the pelvic area, in the middle of the crease where the leg joins the trunk of the body (along the underwear line). In addition to improving fertility, this point helps to relieve menstrual and abdominal cramps in women; it also helps to relieve impotence in men.

Stomach 36

Apply pressure four finger widths below the kneecap, one finger width outside the shinbone. (If you are on the correct spot, a muscle should flex as you move your foot up and down.) In addition to improving fertility, this point helps to build overall vitality and ease fatigue. It also helps relieve impotence in men.

ACUPRESSURE POINTS ON THE INSIDE OF THE FOOT

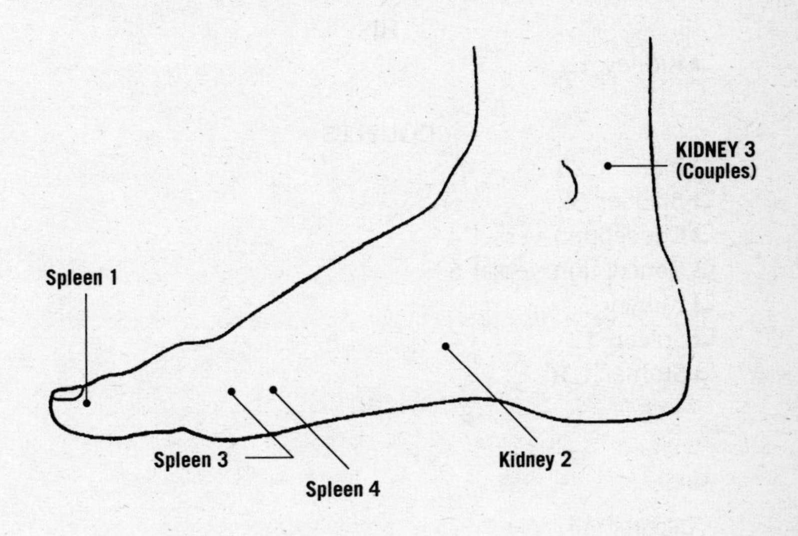

FERTILITY CHECKLIST

HERS

- ❑ Conception vessel 3
- ❑ Governing vessel 23
- ❑ Large intestine 4
- ❑ Spleen 6
- ❑ Spleen 8
- ❑ Spleen 10

HIS

- ❑ Kidney 1

COUPLES

- ❑ Bladder 23
- ❑ Bladder 32
- ❑ Conception vessel 4
- ❑ Conception vessel 6
- ❑ Kidney 3
- ❑ Spleen 12
- ❑ Stomach 36

7

Mind-Body Connection: Fertile Ideas to Boost Your Fertility

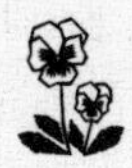

Infertility can cause stress, and stress can cause infertility. Couples who have tried unsuccessfully to conceive a child know firsthand the emotional and physical stress of impaired fertility, but they may not be aware that the stress itself may be contributing to the problem.

Stress inhibits fertility by interfering with the brain's production of reproductive hormones. In the brain, the hypothalamus regulates emotions, appetite, and temperature, and it orchestrates the flow and timing of the reproductive hormones. The hypothalamus is keenly sensitive to all kinds of tensions. Stress, due to anything from travel to job loss to infertility testing itself, can change the way the hypothalamus does its job. In turn, any problem with these hormones can interfere with ovulation and implantation.

Stress can also lower testosterone levels and impair a man's sperm production, in addition to reducing his interest in sex. The adrenaline released during times of stress can decrease blood flow to a man's testes. One study found that sperm production actually stopped in some men facing the death sentence. Other studies have found that the process of undergoing fertility treatment can inhibit a man's sperm production, even if his partner is the one being treated for a reproductive problem.

Researchers estimate that less than 5 percent of infertility is directly related to psychological or emotional factors. Still, evidence suggests that reducing stress can increase a couple's chances of conceiving a child. One study of nurses at the University of Mississippi Medical Center in Jackson found that stress management skills—including deep breathing, meditation, guided imagery, and visualization—helped couples conceive. A group of patients facing in vitro fertilization spent two sessions learning various relaxation techniques. Afterward, 28 percent of the couples in the trained group conceived during their first attempt at in vitro fertilization, compared to just 6 percent of the couples who conceived without practicing stress management. In another study, one out of three infertile women who participated in a relaxation-response-based behavioral treatment program became pregnant within six months.

The Stress Response

When faced with stress, the body kicks into the so-called fight or flight response, which involves a number of biochemical changes that happen in preparation for dealing with danger. In evolutionary terms, this high-intensity state made sense because quick bursts of energy were required to fight off predators or flee a dangerous situation. Of course, in our daily lives we face fewer of these life-or-death threats, but the modern world remains full of different stressors, such as financial worries, health concerns, deadline pressures, and relationship problems. When confronted with these contemporary stressors, our bodies respond in much the same way as our prehistoric ancestors once did.

In the body, any stressor—either real or imagined—triggers an alarm in the hypothalamus in the midbrain. The hypothalamus then shifts into overdrive, warning the body that it must prepare for an emergency. As a result, your heart races, your breathing speeds up, your muscles tense, your metabolism kicks into high gear, and your blood pressure soars. Your blood concentrates in your muscles, leaving your hands and feet cold and your muscles ready for action. Your senses become more acute: Your hearing becomes sharper and your pupils dilate. You're ready for action.

As part of the intricate system of stress response, your body also releases adrenaline, epinephrine, cortisol, and other chemicals that inhibit the immune system and interfere with the release of reproductive hormones. While not harmful in short bursts, these biochemical responses can cause serious health problems if the stress continues for long periods of time. Chronic stress can elevate blood pressure (causing hypertension); it can cause muscle tension (resulting in headaches and digestive disorders); and it can suppress the immune system (leaving an individual susceptible to a wide range of serious diseases).

Fortunately, the stress response can be reversed easily. Your body begins to relax as soon as your brain receives the signal that the danger has passed and it's safe to calm down. About three minutes after the brain cancels the emergency signals to the central nervous system, the panic messages cease and the body begins to relax. Your heart rate and breathing gradually slow down, and your other systems return to their normal levels.

Problems with fertility are certainly not all in your head, but it appears that you can use your head to help enhance your fertility. And, in addition to boosting the odds of conception, stress management skills can help to decrease anxiety, depression, and fatigue, and increase energy, stamina, and well-being.

COUPLES

Enjoy a Good Orgasm

Satisfying sex helps relieve physical tension and stimulate hormone production, both of which can jump start your fertility. Researchers have found that for some people the tension-easing power of a single orgasm can be as much as twenty times more powerful than a dose of a tranquilizer like Valium or Xanax.

Join a Support Group

Joining a support group for couples with impaired fertility increases the chances of conception. It isn't clear whether the benefit comes from the emotional support offered by people in the same situation, or from the fact that the couples have a chance to share practical information on fertility treatments and physicians. Whatever the cause, a study at the University of Massachusetts found that 71 percent (thirty out of forty-two) of infertile couples who participated in a support group eventually became pregnant, compared to 25 percent (twelve out of forty-eight) of those couples who did not join a support group.

Don't Adopt a Child Because You Think It Will Help You Conceive

Many people believe that they will conceive a biological child after they adopt because they will no longer feel stress about conception. There is no truth to the conception-after-adoption myth. Over the past twenty years, repeated studies have found that the frequency of conception among adoptive parents is exactly the same as it is among parents who do not adopt. Of course, adoption offers the opportunity to have children for many couples who may never be able to have biological children. For more information on adoption, consult the organizations listed on page 179.

Practice Stress Relief Techniques

No matter how much stress you're under, you can learn to relax and reverse the stress response by using various mind-body techniques. Studies have shown that well-trained individuals have the ability to use mind-body techniques to voluntarily lower their blood pressure and heart rate, alter their brainwave activity, reduce blood sugar levels, and ease muscle tension. With practice you, too, can put mind over stress and use the following techniques to relax and improve your chances of conceiving a child.

Biofeedback Biofeedback involves training yourself to use your mind to voluntarily control your body's internal systems. Almost anyone can learn biofeedback, but it takes practice. It's easy to get stressed out, but much more difficult to learn to relax and control the precise effect of mind over body.

To learn the skill, you must be able to measure your physical state. To do this, you attach electrodes to various parts of your body to measure your heart rate, breathing, perspiration, pulse, blood pressure, temperature, muscle tension, and brainwave patterns. A small machine on the other end of the wires displays the data, usually in the form of pictures, graphic lines, or audible beeps. Using this information, you can literally watch yourself relax or grow more tense.

You can actually learn to control your body's internal processes by carefully studying the measurable changes in your body as you relax and change your thought patterns. Once you learn to adjust your physical state to promote relaxation, you can do it without all the equipment.

If you'd like to try biofeedback, ask your physician for a referral to an outpatient clinic or look for biofeedback centers listed in the phone book. Before making an appointment, ask about fees and whether the training will be covered by your health insurance plan. For a referral, you can also contact the Association for Applied Psychophysiology and Biofeedback, 10200 West 44th Avenue, Suite 304, Wheat Ridge, CO 80033; (303) 422-8436; or the Biofeedback Certification Institute of America, 10200 West 44th Avenue, Suite 310, Wheat Ridge, CO 80033; (303) 420-2902.

BREATHING Deep breathing helps to relax the body and quiet the mind. Unfortunately, when stressed most people don't breathe right: Instead of inhaling deeply and drawing in plenty of oxygen, they take shallow, rapid, weak breaths, filling only the top part of the lungs. This so-called chest breathing, or thoracic breathing, fails to adequately oxygenate the blood, making it more difficult to manage stress. A better way of breathing is abdominal breathing, or diaphragmatic breathing. Abdominal breathing draws air deeply into the lungs, allowing the chest to fill with air and the belly to rise and fall. Newborn babies and sleeping adults practice abdominal breathing, though most adults lapse into chest breathing during their waking hours.

To relieve stress, become aware of your breathing and inhale more fully. You will immediately be able to feel the muscle tension and stress melt away in response to the improved oxygenation in your tissues. Concentrated, deep breathing can help calm you and relieve stress at any time and in any situation. Of course, don't overdo it or you will hyperventilate. If you experience shortness of breath, heart palpitations, or a feeling that you can't get enough air when practicing deep breathing (the symptoms of hyperventilation), stop immediately and return to your regular breathing pattern.

MASSAGE Massage offers a hands-on way of reducing stress. The technique—which involves soothing touch of the muscles, soft tissues, and ligaments of the body—stimulates blood circulation, slows the heart rate, and lowers blood pressure. It also stimulates the production of disease-fighting antibodies. Studies have found that massage reduces anxiety and stress-related hormones better than other muscle-relaxation techniques. And, instead of making you feel drowsy, it can actually increase your alertness.

You can learn massage techniques yourself, either by checking out a book from a local library or by taking a class. Consider couple's massage, which is good for promoting relaxation, building intimacy, and getting both of you in the mood. You might also consider consulting a massage therapist, who should know a variety of techniques. Most states require licensing of massage therapists; if your state doesn't have licensing, look for a therapist with certification from a professional organization. For information on state licensing requirements and a list of certified massage therapists in your area, call the National Certification Board for Therapeutic Massage and Bodywork at (800) 296-0664. You can also contact the American Massage Therapy Association, 820 Davis Street, Suite 100, Evanston, IL 60201, (708) 864-0123; or the American Oriental Bodywork Therapy Association, Glendale Executive Campus, 1000 White Horse Road, Vorhees, NY 08043, (609) 782-1616.

MEDITATION Though there are many different forms or traditions, meditation basically involves focusing your complete attention on one thing at a time. If you haven't tried it, meditation can be harder than it sounds: The mind tends to wander, and it can be a real challenge to maintain concentration when faced with a barrage of distracting thoughts.

Meditation relieves stress because it is impossible to feel tense or angry when your mind is focused somewhere else. You can't experience negative thoughts—or the physiological responses to those thoughts—if your mind is tuned in to a neutral stimulus.

Studies back up the idea that meditation promotes relaxation. Research done back in 1968 at Harvard Medical School found that when people practiced transcendental meditation (a type of mantra meditation) they showed physiological signs of deep relaxation: Their heart rate and breathing slowed, their oxygen consumption dropped by 20 percent, their blood lactate levels dropped, their skin resistance to electrical current increased, and their brainwave patterns showed greater alpha wave activity.

To experience the relaxing benefits of meditation, find a quiet place where you are not apt to be interrupted. Sit in a firm chair with your back as straight as possible, or lie down flat on your back on the ground. Then try one of the three basic types of meditation:

- *Mantra meditation* involves repeating—either aloud or silently—a word (such as "peace" or "calm"), a syllable (such as "ommmm"), or a group of words (such as "safe and sound" or "I'm okay") each time you breathe out.
- *Gazing meditation* involves focusing both your attention and your gaze on an object such as a candle flame, a stone, or a flower. The object should be

about one foot away from your face. Gaze at it rather than stare, keeping your eyes relaxed. Don't try to think about the object in words, just look at it without judgment.

* *Breathing meditation* involves focusing on the rise and fall of your breath. Draw a deep breath, focusing on the inhalation, the pause before you exhale, the exhalation, and the pause before you inhale. When you exhale, say to yourself "one." Each time you complete a breath and exhale, count again, one through four, then start over with one. The counting helps clear your mind of other thoughts.

No matter which type of meditation you choose, begin your session with a few minutes of deep breathing. When random thoughts enter your mind during your meditation time (as they almost certainly will) don't become anxious; just accept the thoughts and let them pass through your mind without notice or response. Start by meditating for five to ten minutes once or twice a day, then work up to fifteen to twenty minutes.

For more information on meditation, refer to books in the library, take a class from a local recreation center or fitness facility, or practice using instructional tapes. You might also contact one of the following organizations:

Cambridge Insight Meditation Center
331 Broadway
Cambridge, MA 02139
(617) 491-5070

Foundation for Human Understanding
P.O. Box 1009
Grants Pass, OR 97526
(503) 597-4360

Mind/Body Medical Institute
110 Francis Street, Suite 1A
Boston, MA 02215
(617) 632-9525

Stress Reduction Clinic
University of Massachusetts Medical Center
55 Lake Avenue, North
Worcester, MA 01655
(508) 856-2656

Zen Center
300 Page Street
San Francisco, CA 94102
(415) 863-3136

PROGRESSIVE RELAXATION Progressive relaxation can produce a profound feeling of calm as you systematically remove the stress from your body. Start by lying on your back on the floor, with your legs flat and your arms loose at your sides. Close your eyes and breathe deeply.

Once you are reasonably calm, begin to systematically tense and relax every muscle in your body. Start with your feet: Tense the muscles in your feet for thirty seconds or so, then relax, allowing your feet to feel heavy and relaxed. Then move on to your calves, thighs, abdomen, buttocks, hands, forearms, upper arms, shoulders, and face. When you finish, your muscles should feel soothed and relaxed. Lie quietly and enjoy the feeling of complete relaxation.

VISUALIZATION To relieve stress, use your imagination. Visualization—also known as guided imagery—builds on the idea that you are what you think you are. If you think anxious thoughts, your muscles will grow tense; if you think sad thoughts, your brain biochemistry will change and you will become unhappy. And, more importantly, if you think soothing, positive thoughts, you will relax and develop a more positive outlook.

To experience the relaxation of visualization, sit down in a comfortable position or lie on the floor in a quiet, dimly lit room. Tense all of your muscles at once and hold for thirty seconds. Relax every muscle and allow all the tension to drain from your body. Continue to inhale and exhale slowly and fully.

Once your muscles have relaxed, you can begin the visualization or imagery. First, concentrate on your breathing, feeling the regular rhythm of each breath and clearing your mind of all thoughts. Then imagine that you are in a peaceful setting, such as lying in the warm sun on a sandy beach or strolling down a country road on a cool October afternoon. Get all your senses involved in your image: Smell the ocean mist, hear the leaves crunch under your feet. The more specific your fantasy, the more real it will seem. And the more real it seems, the more you will relax. Enjoy this "escape" for about twenty minutes. When you return to your body and get on with the challenges of the day, you will probably feel much more relaxed and refreshed.

For more information on visualization, contact the Mind-Body Medical Institute, New Deaconess Hospital, Harvard Medical School, Boston, MA 02215, (617) 632-9530; or the Academy for Guided Imagery, P.O. Box 2070, Mill Valley, CA 94942, (800) 726-2070.

YOGA Yoga promotes relaxation while at the same time strengthening and stretching the muscles. This form of exercise combines deep breathing with systematically moving the body into a series of postures or positions. It can be very gentle and noncompetitive, but yoga isn't easy. It requires significant endurance, strength, and flexibility. Since it works every muscle group, weaknesses can be identified easily, allowing you to target areas that may need special attention.

There are six main types of yoga; the two most common in the United States are hatha yoga and tantra yoga. (Hatha yoga is what most people think of when they mention yoga.) When practicing hatha yoga, you concentrate on your breathing while assuming a series of physical postures, moving between them slowly and with concentration. Tantra yoga is more meditative and involves the elaborate use of rituals. Both forms build physical strength and relieve stress.

For background on yoga postures and practicing the technique, check out a book on yoga from your local library, take a class at a local "Y" or recreation facility, or rent a yoga video. For professional assistance, look in the Yellow Pages under "yoga" or contact the Integral Yoga Institute, 227 West 13th Street, New York, NY 10011, (212) 929-0586.

FERTILITY CHECKLIST

COUPLES

❑ Have an orgasm.
❑ Join a fertility support group.
❑ Don't adopt a child because you think it will help you conceive.
❑ Practice stress management, including:

- Biofeedback
- Deep breathing
- Massage
- Meditation
- Progressive relaxation
- Visualization
- Yoga

8

Lifestyle: Keys to Conception

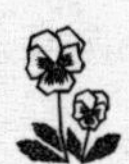

To conceive a child is a remarkable feat. Think about it: It requires precise timing, exquisite hormonal balance, overall good health—and perhaps a touch of divine intervention. While some of these factors are beyond your control, how you live and how you treat your body can have an impact on your overall health and your fertility. That goes both for how you behave now and for what you may have done—or not done—in the past.

HERS

Lose Weight Gradually

Your brain chemistry affects your fertility, and a sudden drop in body weight can throw off the release of gonadotropin-releasing hormone by the hypothalamus in the brain. Crash diets and the corresponding shift in weight can confuse the body's hormone production, possibly resulting in infertility.

If you are overweight, try to lose weight, if possible. Ideally, you should not try to get pregnant until you lose the weight and give your body a chance to adjust to your new physique. Take at least one month of dieting for each six or seven pounds you want to lose (or gain). After reaching your target weight, wait six to eight weeks to give your hormone levels a chance to stabilize before trying to get pregnant. (More under Couples.)

Exercise—But Not Too Much

Regular exercise can help keep you lean and fit, but excessive exercise can keep you from having a baby. If your body fat level dips too low, you may stop ovulating. Or, if you work out more than an hour a day, you may disrupt the timing of your reproductive hormones.

One study found that women who exercised vigorously for more than an hour a day were more likely to experience infertility. Researchers speculate that the endorphins—the feel-good chemicals released during exercise—may alter a woman's prolactin levels, interrupting the timing of ovulation. Don't use the information as an excuse to turn flabby, just exercise in moderation.

Moderation means different things to different women. Strive to work out at least twenty to thirty minutes three times per week, but not more than sixty minutes six times per week. Choose any activity that you enjoy, even running or jogging (unless you have had a problem with miscarriage or your gynecologist recommends against it).

Limit Your Use of Caffeine

It appears that the less caffeine you consume, the more likely you are to get pregnant. Research done at the National Institutes of Health show that drinking as little as one five-ounce cup of coffee—or other foods with the equivalent 115 milligrams of caffeine—can halve your chances of becoming pregnant in any given month compared to women who do not consume caffeine. Another study found that one caffeinated soft drink per day caused the same 50 percent decrease in conception. While not all women seem to respond to restricting caffeine consumption, it can't hurt to give it a try. You can substitute decaffeinated beverages or herbal teas, if you wish.

How Much Caffeine?

Food	*Portion*	*Caffeine (mg)*
Chocolate		
baking, unsweetened	1 ounce	58
chocolate chips (semisweet)	1/4 cup	14
milk chocolate	1 ounce	5 to 10
Cocoa		
hot cocoa mix	1 ounce	5
unsweetened cocoa powder	1 tablespoon	12
Coffee		
brewed	6 ounces	105 to 165
brewed decaf	6 ounces	2 to 5
instant	1 teaspoon	57 to 66
instant decaf	1 teaspoon	2
Soft drinks		
Cola (diet or regular)	12 ounces	35 to 50
Tea		
brewed for three minutes	6 ounces	36
instant	1 teaspoon	31

Note: Many pain relievers also contain caffeine, often 30 milligrams per tablet or more. Alertness tablet typically contain 100 to 200 milligrams per tablet.

Be Wary of Antibiotics

Antibiotics do a tremendous job of killing disease-causing bacteria, but unfortunately they can't differentiate the good bacteria from the bad. As a result, after taking a course of antibiotics, many women develop vaginal yeast infections. Often the culprit is an overgrowth of *Candida*, a type of yeast that leaves the vagina inhospitable to sperm.

To help restore the good bacteria as quickly as possible, try eating yogurt containing live acidophilus cultures or take acidophilus tablets (available at health food stores). You might also drink acidophilus milk, available in many grocery stores. While some health care practitioners may even suggest you insert plain yogurt directly in the vagina, if you are trying to get pregnant you should not put anything containing bacteria inside your vagina.

Give Up Breast-feeding

If you have already had a child and you are breast-feeding, you may need to stop nursing to conceive your next child. Women who do not breast-feed often find that their menstrual cycles return four to ten weeks after childbirth. However, nursing mothers may not ovulate for a year or more, depending on the baby's feeding patterns.

Each time your baby nurses, the brain suppresses the hormone that triggers ovulation. In most cases, ovulation will resume when the baby goes more than four hours between feedings during the day and more than six hours at night. Keep in mind that breast-feeding is not a reliable method of birth control. Ovulation can occur irregularly during nursing, and you may release one egg before experiencing your first menstrual period.

HIS

Wear an Athletic Cup During Sporting Events

Your testicles need to be handled with care. They contain a delicate collection of tiny tubes, ducts, and vessels that can be damaged or scarred by trauma. So, if you're planning to engage in sports that can lead to accident or injury, be sure to wear a protective cup.

Get Off Your Bike

Cycling may be great for physical conditioning, but it's not so great for babymaking. Researchers at the University of Southern California School of Medicine found that cyclists who pedaled one hundred miles a week or more often suffered from "biker's impotence," a condition characterized by difficulty in getting and maintaining an erection for a day or two after biking. The thrusting and banging of the groin against the bicycle seat while pedaling can damage the nerves and arteries in the genital area. To avoid this problem, rise from your bike and support your weight with your legs periodically, or scale back on your riding during the times you are trying to get pregnant.

Keep Your Testicles Cool

The human body is designed to keep the testicles cool. In fact, the scrotal sac is housed outside the body so that the testicles can remain about two degrees cooler than the core body temperature. (The scrotal sac normally keeps the testes at between 94 and 96 degrees F.) Evidence suggests that if the temperature of the testicles rises above 96 degrees F, sperm production and motility is impaired.

In some cases, lowering the scrotal temperature can help make an infertile man into a father. To keep things cool, try the following:

- Avoid hot tubs and saunas.
- Wear boxers rather than briefs or tight bikini underwear. Tight undergarments may heat things up—and not in a way that will enhance your chances of getting pregnant.
- Avoid wearing synthetic fibers during exercise.

Lycra shorts can trap the heat, especially during a workout.

- Exercise, but avoid workouts that heat the testicles. Rowing machines, cross-country ski machines, treadmills, and jogging are the worst culprits when it comes to overheating. Swimming and yoga are good alternatives. After exercise, allow your testicles to hang free and cool off.
- If possible, avoid occupations that keep you in the heat. For example, welding or boiler maintenance operators can work in environments that routinely reach a sperm-killing 120 degrees F.
- Try a cold water treatment. One study found that spraying the scrotum with cool water for two minutes in the morning and evening improved sperm counts in half the men studied.

Give Yourself Time to Recover from Illness

Your body produces about 50 million sperm each day, but it takes about three months for those sperm to be ready for action. It takes about seventy-eight days for sperm to be produced and twelve days more for them to mature. Any kind of viral illness with a fever—even a bad cold—can lower sperm counts for the full three months. The medications you take to treat an illness can also interfere with sperm production. If you have a normal or high sperm count, illness may not lower your sperm count enough to interfere with conception. But if your sperm count is more modest, it may be enough to cause temporary infertility. So be patient; give your sperm time to bounce back after an illness.

Take Steps to Manage Diabetes

Diabetes can wreak havoc on your body—and your sex life. The disease can damage sperm production, and it can cause progressive damage to the blood vessels and nerves in the penis, sometimes resulting in impotence. An estimated 22 to 55 percent of all diabetic men are impotent. Some—but not all men—regain their potency when they bring the illness under control, either by exercising and losing weight or by taking supplemental insulin. To protect your fertility, consult your doctor and take steps to control the illness if you are diabetic.

Find Out if You've Had Mumps—and Get the Vaccine if You Haven't

Mumps is a virus that can cause infertility if it reaches the testicles of a male who has passed puberty; severe cases can damage tissue before puberty as well. (Most childhood cases of mumps do not impair fertility.) Not every case leads to sterility; in roughly half the cases, the virus does not damage the testicles. Other times only one testicle is damaged and the other can compensate.

Fortunately, only about 18 percent of mumps cases occur in men during or past puberty, and in 70 percent of those cases, the virus infects only one testicle. Even if both testicles are affected, when properly treated the disease can usually be stopped before it damages both testicles. In fact, only 5 percent of men who contract mumps become permanently sterile.

If you have not had mumps, talk to your doctor about having a vaccine against the disease.

Treat Varicocele

A varicocele is a varicose vein in the spermatic cord inside the scrotum. These enlarged veins (like those that can form on the backs of the legs) may cause infertility in some men by increasing the temperature inside the testicles. Most varicoceles form above the left testicle in one of the vessels that transport blood from the groin back to the heart.

Varicoceles form deep inside the testicles. While the affected vein cannot be seen, in many cases it can be felt. The condition is said to feel like "a bag of worms" over the top of the testicles. The condition is not painful; in fact, about 8 percent of all men have them, often without experiencing infertility or other problems. However, researchers have found that the condition in roughly 30 to 40 percent of infertile men, and fully 80 percent of those with varicocele have abnormal sperm profiles.

A varicocele can be tied off surgically. In most cases sperm production improves three to six months after the procedure, and in some men up to a year later. About half of all men who undergo treatment regain their fertility following the surgery.

What Is "Normal" Anyway?

It only takes a single sperm to fertilize an egg, but millions of the little swimmers are present in the ejaculate of fertile men. A normal sperm count includes at least 20 million sperm cells per milliliter of ejaculate, or approximately 150 million to 200 million per ejaculation.

Typically, at least half those sperm are "motile," or moving forward, rather than swimming in circles. And at least 40 to 50 percent should be normally shaped. Ideally you want to have both quality and quantity when it comes to sperm, but to protect your fertility, it is better to have fewer high-quality sperm than an abundant supply of sub-par sperm.

COUPLES

Try to Reach—and Maintain—a Reasonable Weight

You may not need another reason to worry about your weight, but evidence suggests that being too fat—or too thin—can affect your fertility. In men, being overweight can cause fertility problems because the testicles become surrounded by fatty tissue, making testicular temperatures rise and sperm counts drop. In women, too much or too little body fat can affect hormone levels and interfere with ovulation.

Women's bodies are particularly susceptible to weight-related fertility problems because women's fat cells are like tiny estrogen manufacturing plants. While some estrogen is produced in the ovaries, 30 percent of the body's supply—and 80 percent during certain points of your menstrual cycle—comes from the fat cells. The typical body fat for a fertile woman is 29 percent; a woman's hormonal system can shut down and she can become infertile if her body fat is more than 10 to 15 percent above or below normal. One study of 276 infertile women with ovulatory dysfunction found that 6 percent of the women had problems because they were overweight, and 6 percent because they were underweight.

Underweight women are often undernourished and

have borderline vitamin and mineral deficiencies. Ultra-thin women often stop having their periods. Also, women who lose 10 to 15 percent of their total body weight (or one-third of their body fat) may stop having periods temporarily. Fortunately, weight gain often helps these women regain their fertility: One study of twenty-nine infertile women (each no more than 91 percent of her ideal body weight) found that those who were able to reach 95 to 100 percent of their ideal weight regained normal ovulation. Within one to three years, twenty-four of twenty-six of these now normal-weight women had become pregnant. Ideally, underweight women who have suffered from amenorrhea (absence of periods) should follow a balanced diet for three or four months after they resume menstruating before they try to conceive.

On the opposite end of the scale, obese women (those more than 20 percent above their ideal weight) produce too much estrogen, which then strains the liver as it tries to break down the excess levels of hormone. The high levels of estrogen also disrupt the hormone system that tells the egg follicle to mature. In fact, oral contraceptive pills take advantage of this hormone response by creating an artificial hormone imbalance. Obese women require higher doses of hormones to induce ovulation than their lean counterparts.

So, how much should you weigh? Your bathroom scale can tell you how much or how little you weigh, but not how fat you are. To assess your body fat, you can calculate your body mass index, or BMI. While bone structure and muscle development can influence accuracy, this method tends to be more reliable than a weight table, and it is accurate enough to give you an idea of whether you have a weight problem that may interfere with conception. Use the following formula:

$$\frac{\text{BMI} = (\text{Weight in Pounds} \times 705) \div \text{Height in Inches}}{\text{Height in Inches}}$$

For example, for a five-foot, seven-inch woman (sixty-seven inches) weighing 135 pounds, the formula would be:

$$\frac{\text{BMI} = (135 \times 705) \div 67}{67} = 21$$

- If your BMI is 19 or less, you are underweight and may need to gain weight to enhance your fertility.
- If your BMI is 20 to 25, you are within your healthy weight range and your weight should not cause a fertility problem.
- If your BMI is 26 to 27, you are somewhat over-

weight, but your weight should not inhibit your fertility;

- If your BMI is 27.5 to 30, you should lose weight before getting pregnant.
- If your BMI is above 30, your weight may be affecting your fertility—as well as your overall health. You need to take steps to gradually lose weight, following a low-fat, high-fiber diet rich in fresh vegetables and fruits.

Where you put those extra pounds also matters. Fat around the middle (the "apple" body shape) is worse for your health than fat around the hips and thighs (the "pear" body shape). A recent study of five-hundred healthy female patients in the Netherlands found that "apples" were only half as likely to get pregnant as "pears." In addition, a waist-to-hip ratio of more than 0.8 for women or more than 1.0 for men is associated with increased risk of heart disease. To calculate your shape, measure your waist at its narrowest point and your hips at their widest, then divide the waist measurement by the hip measurement.

Quit Smoking

You already know that smoking is hazardous to your health. You already know it can cause lung cancer, car-

The Fertility Diet

To lose weight—but not too fast—consume about fifteen hundred calories a day, with an emphasis on low-fat foods that enhance fertility. (Review the foods listed in Chapter 3, "Nutrition and Nutrition Supplements," for a detailed list of foods that promote fertility.) The following food suggestions (prepared using low-fat cooking techniques) may also help:

BREAKFAST

- Orange juice
- Banana OR grapefruit OR orange
- Whole-grain cereal with soy milk OR one-egg omelet containing red pepper and low-fat cheese

LUNCH

- Skim milk
- Turkey sandwich on whole-wheat bread with a single slice of low-fat cheese OR avocado salad
- Green leafy salad
- Yogurt

DINNER

- Fish (twice a week), chicken (twice a week), tofu (twice a week), red meat or organ meat (once a week)—three ounce serving
- Green vegetable
- Brown rice OR new potatoes OR legumes (three times a week), yellow vegetable (four times a week)
- Citrus fruit

SNACKS

- Citrus fruits
- Nuts: hazelnuts, cashews, peanuts, walnuts, soy nuts

diovascular disease, and a number of other serious health problems. But you may not be aware that it can also make it more difficult for you to get pregnant.

If you are among the one in three men or women of childbearing age who smoke cigarettes, do yourself a favor and quit. If you need another reason to kick the habit, consider the evidence supporting a link between smoking and infertility:

✹ Women who smoke have been found to be 3.4 times as likely as nonsmokers to take more than a year to get pregnant, according to a study of 678 women published in the *Journal of the American Medical Association* in 1985.

✹ A 1992 study in the British medical journal *The Lancet* found a 31 percent difference in fertility rates between nonsmoking couples and couples in which both the man and the woman smoked.

✹ Another study found that the fertility of light smokers (less than one pack—twenty cigarettes—a day) was 75 percent of that of nonsmokers; the fertility rate of heavy smokers (more than a pack a day) was 57 percent of that of nonsmokers.

✹ Doctors have known for many years that women who smoke during pregnancy tend to have smaller fetuses and shorter gestation periods than nonsmokers.

✹ Women who smoke during pregnancy miscarry more often. Women who smoke and do become pregnant are almost twice as likely to suffer miscarriage as women who don't smoke, perhaps because smoking reduces estrogen levels.

✹ Even a relatively modest smoking habit can cut short a woman's reproductive life. Women who smoke a half-pack of cigarettes a day experience menopause an average of one year earlier than nonsmokers, and those who smoke one pack enter menopause two years earlier.

✹ In men, as few as sixteen cigarettes a day can decrease sperm count and motility, increase the number of abnormal sperm, and make it less likely that the sperm will fertilize an egg. Evidence also exists that babies born to men who smoke are more likely to have birth defects. The most vulnerable time for smokers is the three-month period before conception when the sperm is being produced.

✹ Smoking saps the body of fertility-enhancing vitamin C, which appears to be one reason for the reduced sperm count among male smokers. Evidence indicates that smokers require at least twice as much vitamin C as nonsmokers. In one study, men with a pack-a-day habit were given either 0 milligrams, 200 milligrams, or 1,000 milligrams of vitamin C. After one month, the men in the 1,000-milligram group had a 140 percent increase in sperm count; those in the 200-milligram group had a 112 percent increase, and the men in the 0-milligram group had no change. More to the point, all the men in the vitamin C group got their partners pregnant within two months, while none of the men in the placebo group had conceived a child. If you smoke, take up to three grams of vitamin C a day (any your body doesn't need will be excreted in your urine).

✻ Be wary of secondhand smoke. Standing in a very smoky room for one hour will be as toxic to your lungs—and your fertility—as directly inhaling ten to fifteen cigarettes.

Stop Drinking Alcohol

Drinking alcohol—even in moderation—can affect the fertility of both women and men. In women, alcohol affects the liver's ability to clear hormonal debris, disrupting hormone levels and interfering with egg production. While the amount of alcohol required to alter brain chemistry and hormone levels varies from woman to woman, evidence suggests that even moderate drinking can contribute to infertility. A 1994 study involving women who used alcohol moderately (one drink or less per day) found a strong correlation between drinking and ovulatory dysfunction and endometriosis. This was after adjustment for age, cigarette smoking, number of sexual partners, use of an intrauterine device, body mass index, and level of exercise.

In men, drinking three drinks a day can cause endocrine abnormalities, low testosterone levels and sperm counts, and an increase in abnormal sperm. Extreme alcohol use (more than five drinks a day) can cause impotence, as well as a temporary inability to ejaculate if an erection does occur.

Recent studies have found that the babies of fathers who drank as few as two drinks a day in the month prior to conception weighed 6.5 ounces less than the babies of teetotaling fathers. This link had nothing to do with whether the mother drank or smoked.

Don't Use Recreational Drugs

There are plenty of good reasons not to use illegal drugs, and inhibiting fertility is just one of them.

- Marijuana carries all the risks and negative side effects of cigarette smoking—and more. Tetrahydrocannabinol (THC), the primary psychoactive ingredient in marijuana, reduces the size of the uterus and ovaries in women; it lowers hormone levels and disrupts menstruation and ovulation. (Female marijuana smokers are three times more likely than nonusers to have irregular menstrual periods.) In men, marijuana use is linked to lowered sperm counts and chromosomally damaged sperm. Smoking marijuana also decreases the male sex drive.
- Cocaine causes birth defects and can trigger miscarriage by stimulating the nervous system, increasing blood pressure and heart rate, and constricting blood vessels. In men, cocaine can raise the core body temper-

ature and damage sperm; it can also cause hormonal imbalances that affect sperm production.

* Hallucinatory drugs, amphetamines, barbiturates, and narcotics all interfere with hormone levels in both men and women, interfering with ovulation in women and sperm production in men.

Avoid the Use of Unnecessary Prescription and Over-the-Counter Drugs

A number of common prescription and nonprescription drugs can inhibit fertility. Stop taking any medications that aren't absolutely necessary. If you're not sure of the possible impact of a drug you're taking, consult your pharmacist or doctor.

A number of drugs can interfere with fertility, including certain antibiotics, anti-seizure drugs, anti-depressive drugs, anti-hypertensive drugs, cortisone and corticosteriods, and anti-ulcer drugs. Women who are trying to get pregnant should avoid antihistamines and decongestants since they may reduce the flow of fertile mucus. Women should also choose aspirin or acetaminophen instead of ibuprofen, a drug that may disrupt ovulation and implantation of the fertilized egg in the uterus.

If you are taking any prescription medicines, discuss your fertility issues with your doctor. Some of these drugs may inhibit fertility—and some may be dangerous

Call for Help

For more information on overcoming an addiction, consider contacting one of the following organizations:

Alcoholics Anonymous
(212) 870-3400, or check Yellow Pages for local listing

American Lung Association
(800) 586-4872

Center for Substance Abuse Prevention
(800) 843-4971

Cocaine Anonymous
(800) COCAINE; (213) 559-5833

Narcotics Anonymous
(800) 662-4357; (818)780-3951

National Clearinghouse for Alcohol and Drug Information
(301) 468-2600

National Institute on Alcoholism and Drug Abuse
(800) 662-4357; (301) 443-4373

to your baby once you do conceive. As an overall rule of thumb, avoid all medications when you're trying to become pregnant, unless your doctor recommends otherwise.

Say No to Steroids

Both men and women use anabolic steroids—and both men and women have their fertility damaged by the use of these dangerous drugs. Anabolic steroids are sometimes used by athletes for bodybuilding and stamina, but they often trigger changes in the pituitary gland that throw the body's hormone balance dangerously out of whack.

Women should never use bodybuilding steroids under any circumstances. In women, they often cause irreversible hormonal imbalances and reproductive problems. Men shouldn't use them, either. They can cause heart problems, depression, rage, and psychosis, in addition to shrunken testicles and sterility. In most cases, men can regain their fertility when they stop using the drugs; a man should abstain from steroid use for at least three months before trying to get his partner pregnant to give his body a chance to cleanse itself of potentially damaged sperm.

Use Your Computer Safely

First researchers thought computers caused fertility problems, then they decided they didn't, and now they once again suspect that computers contribute to a number of reproductive problems, including infertility, miscarriage, and birth defects.

A recent study of almost sixteen hundred women conducted by the Kaiser-Permanente Medical Group in northern California found that women who worked at a computer video display terminal for more than twenty hours per week had twice as many miscarriages in the first trimester of pregnancy as women who did not use computers. In addition, women who used a computer for just five hours a day were 40 percent more likely than nonusers to have babies born with a congenital birth defect. Another study conducted in Manchester, England, found that women who use computers were more likely to experience menstrual irregularities and a failure to ovulate, compared to women who did not use computers.

Men also need to take steps to reduce their exposure to radiation from computers, since radiation has been linked to lowered sperm count, chromosomal damage to the sperm, and testicle damage.

YOU DON'T HAVE TO THROW AWAY YOUR PC

While radiation exposure from computers can impair your fertility, there are steps you can take to protect your reproductive system:

- Most of the radiation escapes from the transformer at the back of your computer monitor, so avoid standing near the rear of your machine. (Most of the radiation falls off within ten feet of the monitor; you're safe if your monitor faces a wall.)
- Keep the monitor at hand's length (as long as you don't experience eye strain) to minimize your radiation exposure.
- If you work in an office with more than one computer, be sure you do not stand or sit near the side or back of anyone else's computer.
- If you have a choice, use a portable or laptop computer; these computers emit lower levels of radiation.
- Choose a monochrome monitor, if possible. These machines may be less fun to work with, but they emit one-quarter to one-third the radiation that color monitors do.

- Consider buying either a special radiation-free monitor or an accessory to cut radiation exposure. These monitors may cost about $100 more; ask your computer dealer for details.

Minimize Air Travel

If you don't have to fly, stay on the ground. Several studies have found that female flight attendants have higher rates of irregular ovulation, infertility, and miscarriage, compared to their grounded counterparts. In men, high levels of atmospheric radiation may cause decreased sperm count, increased sperm abnormalities, and an increase in immature sperm. Avoid as much air travel as possible, especially in the three to five months before you plan to try to get pregnant.

Avoid Environmental Hazards

When trying to get pregnant, you should do everything possible to avoid exposure to as many environmental toxins as you can. Men should be particularly wary of coming in contact with antimony, arsenic, boron, cadmium, lithium, manganese, and mercury because these metals have been found to kill or deform sperm, cause impotence, cause premature or delayed ejaculation, and decrease the ability to have an orgasm. In women, these metals can cause hormonal and menstrual irregularities, problems with embryo implantation, and miscarriage. In particular, cadmium has been implicated in difficulty with implantation, contributing to the fertility problems among women who smoke. (There are some 30 micrograms of cadmium in a single pack of cigarettes.)

Other common hazardous chemicals you should watch out for include dioxin, polychlorinated biphenyls (PCBs), industrial solvents, formaldehyde, nitrous oxide, herbicides, insecticides, and other pesticides. A 1994 study in the British medical journal *The Lancet* reported that organic farmers had healthier sperm than those farmers who used pesticides and chemical fertilizers. If you're a weekend gardener, avoid using pesticides.

Most fertility problems associated with environmental toxins can be reversed if job changes are made. For more information on occupational and environmental toxins that can cause infertility (as well as other health problems), contact the following organizations:

9 to 5
National Association of Working Women
(216) 566-9308

Environmental Protection Agency
Safe Drinking Water Hotline
(800) 426-4791

National Network to Prevent Birth Defects
(202) 543-5450

National Pesticides Telecommunications Network
(800) 858-7378

Occupational Safety and Health Administration (OSHA)
(800) 356-4674

Avoid X-rays and Ionizing Radiation

Prospective parents should take steps to minimize their exposure to X-rays and other types of ionizing radiation. X-ray technicians, dental assistants, doctors, workers in nuclear plants and food irradiation facilities, as well as others in radiation-related jobs should shield their genital areas with a lead apron when appropriate. And, of course, everyone should avoid unnecessary X-rays.

Minimize Your Exposure to Electromagnetic Fields (EMFs)

They're everywhere: from the alarm clock that wakes you in the morning to the electric blanket you wrap up

Who Is at Risk?

While people in almost any profession can be exposed to dangerous substances, people at great risk include people regularly exposed to:

- Automotive exhaust
- Battery production
- Ceramics, glass, or porcelain production
- Dyeing
- Electroplating
- Fingernail care products
- Fireproofing materials
- Gases used for anesthesia
- Hair care products
- Herbicides
- Insecticides
- Jewelry making
- Leather tanning
- Municipal incinerators
- Nitrous oxide (dentists and hygienists)
- Pesticides
- Photography
- Smelting
- Textile manufacturing
- Welding
- Wood finishing

in at night. All those electric appliances that make our lives easier also bombard us with electromagnetic energy or non-ionizing radiation.

X-rays and nuclear devices use ionizing radiation, a type of energy powerful enough to knock electrons off their cellular orbits (which is what can cause genetic mutations and cancer). Non-ionizing radiation, on the other hand, is much weaker, though evidence suggests that it, too, can cause a range of health problems, including infertility.

The effects on the body of exposure to EMFs is very complex, in part because the subject involves a number of variables (including the frequency, wavelength, intensity, and duration of exposure; a person's size, shape, and position relative to the radiation source; and the part of the body that is being exposed, to name a few). Still, more than a thousand studies worldwide have looked at EMFs, and many have found adverse reproductive effects in both humans and animals.

Some studies date back to the 1940s when researchers found reduced sperm counts in radar operators aboard navy ships. Several more recent studies have found increases in miscarriages in magnetic resonance imaging (MRI) operators. Other studies have found as much as a 50 percent increase in miscarriages among women who slept under electric blankets and in electrically heated water beds, compared with women who slept on a conventional mattress and boxspring.

When you are trying to get pregnant, it makes sense to practice what scientists call "prudent avoidance"—in other words, keep your exposure to a minimum. If you're addicted to your electric blanket, turn it on to heat up the bed before your climb in, then unplug it before snoozing (a current runs through the wires whether it's on or off). Distance yourself from your computer screen, printers, copy machines, fax machines, and other office equipment. (As with computers, most of the radiation comes from the back of the machine.) Likewise, try to keep all electric appliances (such as microwaves, stoves, refrigerators, alarm clocks, televisions) at least an arm's length away. The EMFs fall off rapidly with distance, so just a few feet can make all the difference.

FERTILITY CHECKLIST

HERS

- ❑ Lose weight gradually, or gain weight if necessary.
- ❑ Exercise in moderation.
- ❑ Avoid caffeine.
- ❑ Be wary of antibiotics.
- ❑ Give up breast-feeding.

HIS

- ❑ Wear an athletic cup.
- ❑ Avoid distance biking.
- ❑ Keep your testicles cool:

    - ✺ Avoid hot tubs and saunas.
    - ✺ Wear boxers rather than briefs or bikini underwear.
    - ✺ Avoid wearing synthetic shorts during exercise.
    - ✺ Avoid workouts that heat the testicles.
    - ✺ Avoid high-heat occupations.
    - ✺ Try a cold-water treatment

- ❑ Give your sperm a chance to recover from illness.
- ❑ Manage diabetes.
- ❑ Get a mumps vaccine, if appropriate.
- ❑ Treat varicocele.

COUPLES

- ❑ Maintain a reasonable weight.
- ❑ Quit smoking.
- ❑ Stop drinking alcohol.
- ❑ Don't use recreational drugs.
- ❑ Avoid unnecessary prescription and over-the-counter drugs.
- ❑ Don't use anabolic steroids.
- ❑ Use your computer safely.
- ❑ Minimize air travel.
- ❑ Avoid environmental hazards.
- ❑ Avoid X-rays and radiation.
- ❑ Minimize your exposure to electromagnetic fields.

Resources

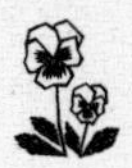

ORGANIZATIONS OF INTEREST

Infertility

American College of Obstetricians and Gynecologists
P.O. Box 96920
409 Twelfth Street, S.W.
Washington, DC 20090-6920
(202) 638-5577

This group can provide a list of board-certified reproductive endocrinologists, as well as consumer information brochures on fertility.

American Self-Help Clearinghouse
Northwest Covenant
25 Pocono Road

Denville, NJ 07834

(201) 625-7101

This group offers phone numbers for support groups on infertility and other topics; it also provides information on how to start a support group.

American Society for Reproductive Medicine

1209 Montgomery Highway

Birmingham, AL 35216-2809

(205) 978-5000

E-mail: asrm@asrm.com

Web site: http://www.asrm.com

This nonprofit organization publishes the monthly journal *Fertility and Sterility* and provides information on infertility and other issues associated with reproductive medicine. A list of infertility specialists is available on request. In addition, a list of patient brochures is included on the Internet site.

Fertility Resource Foundation

877 Park Avenue

New York, NY 10021

(212) 744-5500

This groups offers brochures and information on infertility; there is a fee for some of the materials.

National Infertility Network Exchange
P.O. Box 204
East Meadow, NY 11554
(516) 794-5772
E-mail: nine204@aol.com

This nonprofit organization maintains a national referral service of doctors, lawyers, clinics, donor programs, and other fertility-related resources. The group publishes a bimonthly newsletter, runs support groups, and holds workshops on fertility and adoption.

Reproductive Toxicology Center
2440 M Street, N.W., Suite 217
Washington, DC 20037-1404
(202) 293-5137

This organization operates a database on the effects on reproduction of chronic or acute exposure to thousands of potentially toxic substances. The center serves health care professionals only; if you have a specific question, ask your doctor to call for more information.

RESOLVE, Inc.
1310 Broadway
Somerville, MA 02144-1779
(617) 623-0744

E-mail: resolveinc@aol.com
Web site: http://www.resolve.org

This group provides information, support, and referral to specialists for men and women with infertility problems. The group sponsors local support groups, publishes a newsletter and fact sheets, and makes physician referrals.

Society for Reproductive Endocrinologists, Inc.
1209 Montgomery Highway
Birmingham, AL 35216-2809
(205) 978-5000

This group, which is an affiliate of the American Society for Reproductive Medicine, can provide a list of member doctors; all must be board certified in reproductive endocrinology or have similar qualifications.

In addition, computer users may find the following Usenet newsgroups helpful:

- alt.infertility
- misc.health.infertility

Adoption

National Council for Adoption
1930 Seventeenth Street, N.W.
Washington, DC 20009
(202) 328-1200

This group provides information on adoption, including domestic, international, and special-needs adoptions.

Adoptive Families of America
2309 Como Avenue
St. Paul, MN 55108
(612) 535-4829

This organization provides support and information to adoptive families, and those considering adoption. The group also can provide information on local chapters and support networks.

International Concerns Committee for Children
911 Cypress Drive
Boulder, CO 80303
(303) 494-8333

This group provides information and support for orphan children in many countries. The organization publishes *The Foreign Adoption Report,* an annual listing of foreign adoption resources for U.S. citizens, and also a listing of children available for adoption by U.S. adoptive families.

Nutrition and Nutrition Supplements

If you have special nutritional needs or want help designing a regimen of nutrition supplements to help boost your fertility, you may want to consult a nutrition counselor. For information on finding a qualified nutrition counselor, contact:

American Academy of Nutrition
3408 Sausalito Drive
Corona Del Mar, CA 92625
(800) 290-4226

This group offers referrals to more than four hundred graduates of a fifteen-month program accredited by Distance Education and Training Council of the U.S. Department of Education.

National Institute of Nutritional Education
1010 South Joliet Street, #107
Aurora, CO 80012
(303) 340-2054

This group provides free referrals to 750 certified practitioners who have completed coursework and passed exams on nutrition; practitioners must update their certification annually.

For help with specific questions about nutrition, contact:

Consumer Nutrition Hotline
(sponsored by the American Dietetic Association)
(800) 366-1655

The hotline staff can answer questions and provide free referrals to registered dietitians in your area.

Publications on nutrition are available (some for a fee) from:
American Council on Science and Health
1995 Broadway, Sixteenth Floor
New York, NY 10023-5860
(212) 362-7044

American Institute of Nutrition
9650 Rockville Pike, Suite L4500
Bethesda, MD 20814-3990
(301) 530-7050

Nutrition Action Health Letter
Center for Science in the Public Interest
1875 Connecticut Avenue, N.W., Suite 300
Washington, DC 20009-5728
(202) 332-9111

Society for Nutrition Education
2001 Killebrew Drive, Suite 340
Minneapolis, MN 55425-1882
(612) 854-0035

Herbal Medicine

Herbal medicine is used by many naturopathic physicians and acupuncturists. There is no separate certification or licensing process specifically for practitioners of herbal medicine. Look for a practitioner who is a member of a professional organization, such as the American Herbalists Guild.

For information on herbal medicine and referrals to practitioners in your area, contact:

American Herbalists Guild
P.O. Box 1683
Soquel, CA 95073
(408) 464-2441

Additional publications, newsletters, and books on herbal medicine are available from:

American Botanical Council
P.O. Box 201660
Austin, TX 78720-1660
(512) 331-8868
(800) 373-7105

Herb Research Foundation
1007 Pearl Street, Suite 200
Boulder, CO 80302
(303) 449-2265

Manufacturers of herb mail-order catalogs include:

East Earth Trade Winds
P.O. Box 493151
Redding, CA 96049-3151
(800) 258-6878
(916) 241-6878 in California

Herb-Pharm
P.O. Box 116
William, OR 97544
(541) 846-6262

McZand Herbal Inc.
P.O. Box 5312
Santa Monica, CA 90409
(310) 822-0500

Meridian Traditional Herbal Products
44 Linden Street
Brookline, MA 02146
(800) 356-6003
(617) 739-2636 in Massachusetts

Nature's Way Products, Inc.
10 Mountain Springs Parkway
Springville, UT 84663
(801) 489-1520

Windriver Herbs
P.O. Box 3876
Jackson, WY 83001
(800) 903-HERB

Homeopathy

Homeopathy is practiced by medical doctors (M.D.'s), osteopaths (D.O.'s), naturopaths (N.D.'s), chiropractors (D.C.'s), and dentists (D.D.S.'s). Some states also allow chiropractors, family nurse practitioners, acupuncturists, and physician assistants to obtain licensure.

For an information packet on homeopathy and a directory of practitioners, contact:

National Center for Homeopathy
801 North Fairfax Street, Suite 306
Alexandria, VA 22314
(703) 548-7790

There is a $6 fee for the information packet and directory. The center also publishes the monthly magazine *Homeopathy Today*; cost: $40 a year.

Homeopathic Educational Services
2124 Kittredge Street
Berkeley, CA 94704
(510) 649-0294

This groups charges $8 for a directory of National Center for Homeopathy members, plus a list of homeopathic study groups and manufacturers. Other educational materials are also available.

Manufacturers of homeopathic medicines that offer mail-order catalogs:

Apothecary
5415 Cedar Lane
Bethesda, MD 20814
(301) 530-0800

Apthorp Pharmacy
2201 Broadway at Seventy-Eighth Street
New York, NY 10024
(800) 775-3582
(212) 877-3480

Bailey's Pharmacy
175 Harvard Avenue
Allston, MA 02134
(800) 239-6206
(617) 782-7202

Boericke and Tafel, Inc.
2381 Circadian Way
Santa Rosa, CA 95407
(707) 571-8202

Budget Pharmacy
3001 N.W. Seventh Street
Miami, FL 33125
(800) 221-9772

Dolisos America, Inc.
3014 Rigel Avenue
Las Vegas, NV 89102
(702) 871-7153

Ehrhart and Karl, Inc.
17 North Wabash Avenue
Chicago, IL 60602
(773) 248-5588

Five Elements Center
115 Route 46W
Building D, Suite 29
Mount Lakes, NJ 07046
(201) 402-8510

Hahnemann Pharmacy
828 San Pablo Avenue
Albany, CA 94706
(510) 527-3003

Homeopathic Educational Services
2124 Kittredge Street
Berkeley, CA 94707
(510) 649-0294

Homeopathy Overnight
4111 Simon Road
Youngstown, OH 44512
(800) ARNICA-30

Luyties Pharmacal Company
4200 Laclede Avenue
St. Louis, MO 63108
(800) 325-8080

Santa Monica Homeopathic Pharmacy
629 Broadway
Santa Monica, CA 90401
(310) 395-1131

Standard Homeopathy Company
P.O. Box 61067
154 West 131st Street
Los Angeles, CA 90061
(213) 321-4284

Taylor's Pharmacy
339 South Park Avenue
Winter Park, FL 32789
(407) 644-1025

Washington Homeopathic Pharmacy
4914 Del Ray Avenue
Bethesda, MD 20814
(301) 656-1695

Weleda Pharmacy, Inc.
175 North Route 9W
Congers, NY 10920
(914) 268-8572

Acupressure and Acupuncture

While you can practice acupressure as a self-help technique, you may want to consult a professional if you have additional questions, or if you would like to try acupuncture for a more powerful healing effect. Nationwide, approximately three thousand medical doctors and osteopaths have studied acupuncture and use it as one of the tools in their medical practice. An additional seven thousand naturopaths and other nonphysician healers use acupressure and acupuncture.

Acupuncture and acupressure professionals must meet state licensing or certification requirements in twenty-nine states and the District of Columbia. All states allow medical doctors to practice acupuncture, but only fourteen require physicians to have formal training in it.

If you want to use a physician acupuncturist or acupressurist, look for someone who is a member of the American Academy of Medical Acupuncture. To become a member, a physician must complete at least two hundred hours of acupuncture training and two years experience. Approximately three thousand doctors practice acupuncture in the United States today, but only about five hundred of them are AAMA members. For more information or a referral, contact:

American Academy of Medical Acupuncture (AAMA)
5820 Wilshire Boulevard, Suite 500
Los Angeles, CA 90036
(213) 937-5514

If you're interested in seeing a nonphysician acupuncturist or acupressurist, make sure he or she has been certified by the National Commission for the Certification of Acupuncturists. (A certified member can use the title Diplomate of Acupuncture, indicated by the initials Dipl. Ac. after his or her name.) To become certified, an acupuncturist must pass both a written and a practical exam; to be eligible to take the exams, he or she must be licensed, must have at least two years of training or must have worked as an apprentice acupuncturist for at least four years. For more information or to confirm certification of a particular acupuncturist or acupressurist, contact:

National Certification Commission of Acupuncture and Oriental Medicine (NCCA)
P.O. Box 97075
Washington, DC 20090
(202) 232-1404

For additional information on acupuncture and acupressure, as well as for a free referral to practitioners in your area, contact:

Acupressure Institute of America
1533 Shattuck Avenue
Berkeley, CA 94709
(800) 442-2232
(415) 845-1059 in California

American Association for Acupuncture and Oriental Medicine
433 Front Street
Catasauqua, PA 18032-2506
(610) 266-1433

Mind-body Medicine

American Board of Hypnotherapy
16842 Von Karman Avenue, Suite 475
Irvine, CA 92606
(800) 872-9996

This group provides referrals to its ten thousand member practitioners who have been certified and registered by the board.

Biofeedback Certification Institute of America
10200 West 44th Avenue, Suite 304
Wheat Ridge, CO 80033
(303) 420-2902

This group offers free referrals to practitioners of biofeedback therapy. Submit your request in writing with a stamped, self-addressed envelope.

Center for Mind-Body Medicine
5225 Connecticut Avenue, N.W., Suite 414
Washington, DC 20015
(202) 966-7338

This nonprofit educational organization provides information on mind-body healing. The group offers workshops on mind-body techniques to enhance health and to improve fertility. It also offers a directory of local and national practitioners, organizations, and resources to assist you in locating complementary health care information. The directory costs $10.

Holistic Medicine

Holistic medicine is practiced by medical doctors (M.D.'s), osteopaths (D.O.'s), and naturopaths (N.D.'s). These physicians emphasize the treatment of the whole person and encourage personal responsibility for health.

For a national directory of licensed holistic practitioners, contact:

American Holistic Medical Association
4101 Lake Boone Trail, #201
Raleigh, NC 27607
(919) 787-5146

There is a $5 fee for the national referral directory. The association also publishes the magazine *Holistic Medicine* four times a year for its members.

American Holistic Health Association
P.O. Box 17400
Anaheim, CA 92817-7400
(714) 779-6152
E-mail: ahha@healthy.net
Web site: http://www.healthy.net/ahha

The group is a national clearinghouse of self-help resources; it offers resource lists, publishes a newsletter, and sponsors lectures.

Holistic Health Directory and Resource Guide
42 Pleasant Street
Watertown, MA 02172
(617) 926-0200

This is a directory of more than seven thousand alternative practitioners in over one hundred treatment categories nationally. The directory is revised annually. It is available for $5.95 from bookstores, health food stores, or the publisher.

Naturopathy

Most naturopathic physicians are graduates of a four-year postgraduate medical sciences program. Their training includes courses in herbal medicine, nutrition, homeopathy, exercise therapy, acupressure, and acupuncture. In a number of states naturopathic physicians (N.D.'s) must pass a state licensing exam. *Note:* Some people claiming to be trained naturopaths have only taken mail-order training; be sure to inquire about the training of any medical professional you plan to consult.

For a directory of qualified naturopathic physicians and a list of states with licensing requirements, contact the professional organization of licensed naturopathic physicians:

American Association of Naturopathic Physicians
2366 East Lake Avenue East, Suite 322
Seattle, WA 98102
(206) 323-7610

There is a $5 fee for the information packet and national directory of members.

RECOMMENDED READING

Adoption

Adamec, Christine, and William Pierce. *The Encyclopedia of Adoption.* New York: Facts on File, 1991.

Alexander-Roberts, Colleen. *The Essential Adoption Handbook.* Dallas: Taylor Publishing Company, 1993.

Beauvais-Godwin, Laura, and Raymond Godwin. *The Independent Adoption Manual.* Lakewood, N.J.: Advocate Press, 1993.

Bolles, Edmund Blair. *The Penguin Adoption Handbook.* New York: Penguin Books, 1984.

Canepe, Charlene. *Adoption: Parenthood Without Pregnancy.* New York: Henry Holt, 1986.

Elgart, Arty, and Claire Berman. *Golden Cradle: How the Adoption Establishment Works—and How to Make It Work for You.* New York: Citadel Press, 1991.

Gilman, Lois. *The Adoption Resource Book.* New York: Harper & Row, 1992.

Hicks, Randall. *Adopting in America: How to Adopt Within One Year*. Sun City, Calif.: Wordslinger Press, 1996.

Melina, Lois Ruskai. *Making Sense of Adoption: A Parent's Guide*. New York: Harper & Row, 1989.

Michelman, Stanley, and Meg Schneider. *The Private Adoption Handbook*. New York: Villard Books, 1989.

Plumez, Jacqueline Hornar. *Successful Adoption*. New York: Harmony Books, 1982.

Sullivan, Michael R., and Susan Shulz. *Adopt the Baby You Want*. New York: Simon and Schuster, 1990.

van Gulden, Holly, and Lisa M. Bartels-Rabb. *Real Parents, Real Children*. New York: Crossroad, 1993.

Infertility

Becker, Gay. *Healing the Infertile Family*. New York: Bantam, 1990.

Bellina, Joseph, M.D., Ph.D., and Josleen Wilson. *You Can Have a Baby*. New York: Crown, 1985.

Berger, Gary, M.D., and Marc Goldstein, M.D. *The Couple's Guide to Fertility*. New York: Doubleday, 1994.

Boston Women's Health Book Collective. *The New Our Bodies, Ourselves*. New York: Simon & Schuster, 1992.

Cooper, Susan, Ed.D., and Ellen Glazer, LICSW. *Beyond Infertility: New Paths to Parenthood*. Lexington, Mass.: Lexington Books, Macmillan, 1994.

Corson, Stephen L. M.D. *Conquering Infertility: A Guide for Couples*. New York: Prentice-Hall Press, 1990.

Edwards, Margot, ed. *A Stairstep Approach to Fertility*. Freedom, Calif.: Crossing Press, 1989.

Franklin, Robert R., M.D., and Dorothy Kay Brockman. *In Pursuit of Fertility: A Consultation With a Specialist*. New York: Henry Holt & Co., 1990.

Freeman, Sarah, Ph.D., R.N.C., and Vern L. Bullough, Ph.D., R.N. *The Complete Guide to Fertility and Family Planning*. Buffalo, N.Y.: Prometheus Books, 1993.

Glazer, Ellen Sarasohn, and Susan Lewis Cooper. *Without Child: Experiencing and Resolving Infertility*. Lexington, Mass.: D.C. Health, 1988.

Goldfarb, Herbert A., M.D., with Zoe Graves, Ph.D. *Overcoming Infertility*. New York: John Wiley and Sons, 1995.

Hanson, Michelle. *Infertility: The Emotional Journey*. Minneapolis: Deaconess Press, 1994.

Harkness, Carla. *The Infertility Book: A Comprehensive Medical and Emotional Guide*. Berkeley, Calif.: Celestial Arts, 1992.

Karow, William G., M.D., William C. Gentry, Christopher Hsuing, and Andrienne Pope, Ph.D. *A Baby of Your Own: New Ways to Overcome Infertility*. Dallas: Taylor Publishing, 1992.

Kass-Annese, Barbara, R.N., C.N.P., and Hal C. Danzer, M.D. *The Fertility Awareness Handbook: The Natural Guide to Avoiding or Achieving Pregnancy.* Alameda, Calif.: Hunter House, 1992.

Lauersen, Niels H., M.D., Ph.D. and Colette Bouchez. *Getting Pregnant: What Couples Need to Know Right Now.* New York: Fawcett Columbine, 1991.

Levitt, B. Blake. *50 Essential Things to Do When the Doctor Says It's Infertility.* New York: Plume, 1995.

Madaras, Lynda, and Jane Patterson, M.D. *Womancare.* New York: Avon 1984.

Menning, Barbara Eck. *Infertility: A Guide for the Childless Couple.* Englewood Cliffs, N.J.: Prentice-Hall, 1988.

Nachtigall, Robert, M.D. and Elizabeth Mehran. *Overcoming Infertility.* New York: Doubleday, 1991.

Novotny, Pamela Patrick. *What You Can Do About Infertility.* New York: Dell Publishing, 1991.

Pfeiffer, Regina Asaph, and Katherine Whitlock. *Fertility Awareness: How to Become Pregnant When You Want to, and Avoid Pregnancy When You Don't.* Englewood Cliffs, N.J.: Prentice-Hall, 1984.

Raab, Diana, R.N. *Getting Pregnant and Staying Pregnant.* Montreal: Sirdan Publications, 1988.

Robin, Peggy. *How to Be a Successful Fertility Patient.* New York: William Morrow, 1993.

Rosenberg, Helane, Ph.D. and Yakov Epstein, Ph.D. *Get-*

ting Pregnant When You Thought You Couldn't. New York: Warner, 1993.

Rosenthal, Sara. *The Fertility Sourcebook.* Los Angeles: Lowell House, 1995.

Salzer, Linda P. *Surviving Infertility: A Compassionate Guide Through the Emotional Crisis of Infertility.* New York: Harper Perennial, 1991.

Sussman, John R. M.D., and B. Blake Levitt. *Before You Conceive: The Complete Prepregnancy Guide.* New York: Bantam Books, 1989.

Tan, S.L., M.D., H.S. Jacobs, M.D., and M.M. Seibel, M.D. *Infertility: Your Questions Answered.* New York: Birch Lane Press, 1995.

Treiser, Susan, M.D., Ph.D., and Robin K. Levinson. *A Woman Doctor's Guide to Infertility.* New York: Hyperion, 1994.

Weschler, Toni, MPH. *Taking Charge of Your Fertility: The Definitive Guide to Natural Birth Control and Pregnancy Achievement.* New York: Harper Perennial, 1995.

Natural Medicine

Balch, James and Phyllis. *Prescription for Nutritional Healing.* Garden City Park, N.Y.: Avery Publishing Group, 1990.

Bauer, Cathryn. *Acupressure for Everybody.* New York: Henry Holt, 1991.

Carper, Jean. *The Food Pharmacy.* New York: Bantam Books, 1988.

Carper, Jean. *Food—Your Miracle Medicine: How Food Can Prevent and Cure Over 100 Symptoms and Problems.* New York: HarperCollins, 1993.

Castleman, Michael. *The Healing Herbs: The Ultimate Guide to the Curative Power of Nature's Medicines.* New York: Bantam Books, 1991.

Castro, Miranda. *The Complete Homeopathy Handbook.* New York: St. Martin's Press, 1990.

Cummings, S., and D. Ullman. *Everybody's Guide to Homeopathic Medicines.* Los Angeles: J.P. Tarcher, 1984.

Dobelis, Inge N., ed. *Magic and Medicine of Plants.* Pleasantville, N.Y.: Reader's Digest, 1986.

Firebrace, Peter, and Sandra Hill. *Acupuncture: How It Works, How It Cures.* New Canaan, Conn.: Keats Publishing, 1994.

Gach, Michael Reed. *Acupressure's Potent Points.* New York: Bantam Books, 1990.

Griffith, Winter H. *The Complete Guide to Vitamins, Minerals, Supplements, and Herbs.* Tucson: Fisher Books, 1988.

Hallowell, Michael. *Herbal Healing.* Garden City Park, N.Y.: Avery Publishing Group, 1994.

Israel, Richard. *The Natural Pharmacy Product Guide.* Garden City Park, N.Y.: Avery Publishing Group, 1991.

Kowalchik, Claire, and William H. Hylton, eds. *Rodale's Illustrated Encyclopedia of Herbs.* Emmaus, Pa: Rodale Press, 1987.

Kushi, Michio, and Stephen Blauer. *The Macrobiotic Way.* Avery Publishing Group, 1985.

Law, Donald. *The Concise Herbal Encyclopedia.* New York: St. Martin's Press, 1973.

Lockie, Dr. Andrew. *The Family Guide to Homeopathy: Symptoms and Natural Solutions.* New York: Fireside, 1989.

Murray, Michael, N.D., and Joseph Pizzorono, N.D. *Encyclopedia of Natural Medicine.* Rocklin, Calif.: Prima Publishing, 1991.

Olsen, Kristin Gottschalk. *The Encyclopedia of Alternative Health Care.* New York: Pocket Books, 1989.

Reader's Digest Association, ed. by Alma E. Guinness. *Reader's Digest Family Guide to Natural Medicine: How to Stay Healthy the Natural Way.* New York: Reader's Digest, 1993.

Rosenfeld, Isadore, M.D. *Doctor, What Should I Eat? Nutrition Prescriptions for Ailments in Which Diet Can*

Really Make a Difference. New York: Random House, 1995.

Tyler, Varro, Ph.D. *The Honest Herbal.* Binghamton, N.Y.: Pharmaceutical Products Press, 1993.

Weil, Andrew, M.D. *Health and Healing.* Boston: Houghton Mifflin, 1983.

Weil, Andrew, M.D. *Natural Health, Natural Medicine.* Boston: Houghton Mifflin, 1990.

Weiner, Michael. *The Complete Book of Homeopathy.* Garden City Park, N.Y.: Avery Publishing Group, 1989.

Weiss, Gaea and Shandor. *Growing and Using the Healing Herbs.* Emmaus, Pa.: Rodale Press, 1985.

Index

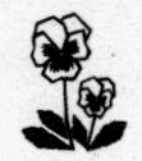

Page numbers in italics indicate sidebars and illustrations

INDEX

Index

About the Author

First and foremost, Winifred Conkling is the mother of two children, Hannah (who was conceived the first month of "trying") and Ella (who took considerably longer and ultimately inspired this book). Once the kids are asleep, Conkling transforms into a freelance writer with extensive experience writing about health and alternative medicine. She is the author of *Stopping Time: Natural Remedies for Aging* (Dell, 1997), *Natural Remedies for Arthritis* (Dell, 1997), *Natural Remedies for Children* (St. Martin's, 1996), *Trade Secrets* (Fireside, 1995), and *Securing Your Child's Future* (Ballantine, 1995), among other books. Her work has been published in a number of national magazines, including *American Health, Consumer Reports, Mademoiselle, McCall's,* and *Reader's Digest*.